Cooling the Flames

Ellis Amdur, M.A., N.C.C., C.M.H.S.
John K. Murphy, JD, MS, PA-C, EFO

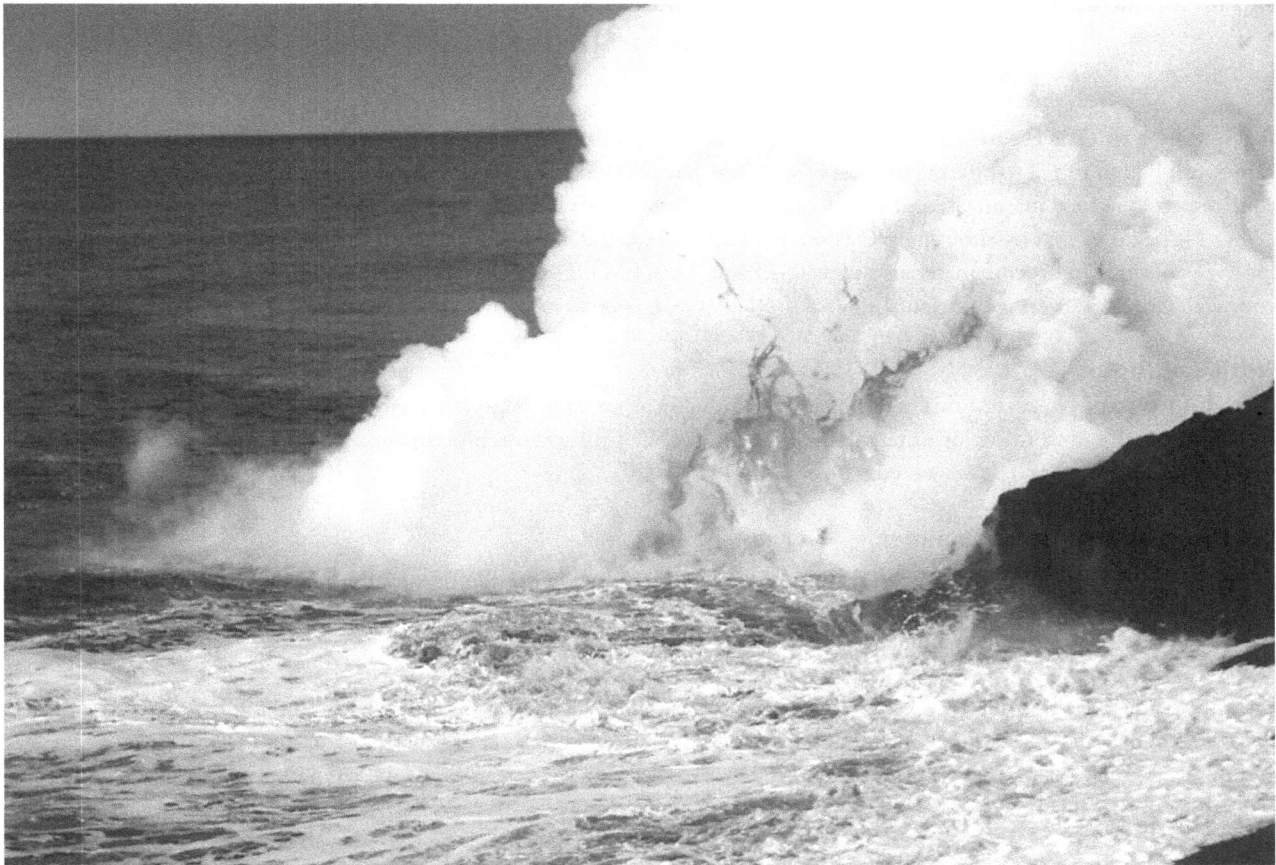

Communication, Control, and De-escalation of
Mentally Ill and Aggressive Patients

A Comprehensive Guidebook for

Firefighters and Emergency Medical Services

An Edgework Book
www.edgework.info

Notes and Notices

COOLING THE FLAMES: Communication, Control, and De-escalation of Mentally Ill and Aggressive Patients
A Comprehensive Guidebook for Firefighters and Emergency Medical Services

By Ellis Amdur, M.A., N.C.C., C.M.H.S. and John K. Murphy, JD, MS, PA-C, EFO © 2015

ISBN: 978-1-950678-06-8

A Message to Our Readers

Edgework is committed to offering the best of what our years of experience and study have taught us. We ask that you express your respect for these intentions and honor our work by adhering strictly to the copyright protection notice you will find below. Please know that by choosing NOT to reproduce these materials, you are supporting our work and making it possible for us to continue to develop materials that will enhance both EMT/Firefighter and public safety. We thank you sincerely for your vigilance in respecting our rights!

Credits
Photographs by: Dreamstime.com
Illustrations by: Shoko Zama
Design: Soundview Design Studio
Cover photograph by: T.J. Takahashi, Wikimedia Commons

Contents

Published Works by Ellis Amdur (and Co-Authors)

Published by Edgework www.edgework.info

COOLING THE FLAMES: Verbal De-escalation of Mentally Ill and Emotionally Disturbed Patients
A Comprehensive Guidebook for Firefighters and Emergency Medical Services
Ellis Amdur & John K Murphy

EVERYTHING ON THE LINE: Calming and De-escalation of Aggressive and Mentally Ill Individuals on the Phone
A Comprehensive Guidebook for Emergency Dispatch (9-1-1) Centers
Ellis Amdur

FROM CHAOS TO COMPLIANCE: Communication, Control, and De-escalation of Mentally Ill, Emotionally Disturbed and Aggressive Offenders
A Comprehensive Guidebook for Parole and Probation Officers
Ellis Amdur & Alan Pelton

GRACE UNDER FIRE: Skills to Calm and De-escalate Aggressive and Mentally Ill Individuals in Outpatient Settings: 2nd Edition
A Comprehensive Guidebook for Health and Social Services Agencies, and Individual Practitioners
Ellis Amdur

GUARDING THE GATES: Calming, Control and De-escalation of Mentally Ill, Emotionally Disturbed and Aggressive Individuals
A Comprehensive Guidebook for Security Guards
Ellis Amdur & William Cooper

IN THE EYE OF THE HURRICANE: Skills to Calm and De-escalate Aggressive and Mentally Ill Family Members: 2nd Edition
Ellis Amdur

SAFE BEHIND BARS: Communication, Control, and De-escalation of Mentally Ill and Aggressive Inmates
A Comprehensive Guidebook for Correctional Officers in Jail Settings
Ellis Amdur, Michael Blake & Chris De Villeneuve

SAFE HAVEN: Skills to Calm and De-escalate Aggressive and Mentally Ill Individuals: 2nd Edition
A Comprehensive Guidebook for Personnel Working in Hospital and Residential Settings
Ellis Amdur

SAFETY AT WORK: Skills to Calm and De-escalate Aggressive and Mentally Ill Individuals
A Comprehensive Guidebook for Corporate Security Managers, Human Resources Staff, Loss Prevention Specialists, Executive Protection, and Others Involved in Threat Management Professions
Ellis Amdur & William Cooper

THE THIN BLUE LIFELINE: Verbal De-escalation of Mentally Ill and Emotionally Disturbed People
A Comprehensive Guidebook for Law Enforcement Officers
Ellis Amdur & John Hutchings

Published by Freelance Academy Press, Inc. www.freelanceacademypress.com

DUELING WITH OSENSEI: Grappling with the Myth of the Warrior Sage, Expanded Edition
Ellis Amdur

HIDDEN IN PLAIN SIGHT: Tracing the Roots of Ueshiba Morihei's Power 2nd Edition
Ellis Amdur

OLD SCHOOL: Essays on Japanese Martial Traditions, Expanded Edition
Ellis Amdur

Fiction
Published by Jet City Comics

CIMARRONIN: A Samurai in New Spain (a graphic novel)
Neal Stephenson, Charles Mann, Mark Teppo & Ellis Amdur

Published by Amazon KDP

THE GIRL WITH THE FACE OF THE MOON
Ellis Amdur

Published Works by John K Murphy

Published by Prentice Hall

LEGAL, POLITICAL & REGULATORY ENVIRONMENT IN EMS

In Gratitude for Expert Critique

The following professionals have closely reviewed this book. With each critique, we corrected errors of fact, added new information, and fine-tuned the manuscript. One of the qualities of a good firefighter or EMT is the understanding that the task supersedes protecting someone's feelings; therefore, we have appreciated all the direct criticism.

All responsibility for this book, however, must lie in our hands. Any errors, in particular, are our responsibility alone. Given that lives can be on the line in work such as this, please do not hesitate to contact us if you believe that any part of this book is inaccurate or needs additional material. We will revise the book, as needed, in future editions. Our thanks to:

Gary L. Aleshire, Jr. is the owner and COO of Future Values, which provides subject matter expert services, organizational efficiency and effectiveness assessments, strategic planning and recommendations, capital project development and established operational performance measure goals systems.

Gary completed his undergraduate and graduate studies from the University of Washington and has attained his Masters in Business Administration with a focus on change management.

He has been involved in the fire service for over 32 years, most recent as Assistant Fire Chief for Snohomish County, Fire District 1 located north of Seattle and prior to, twenty-five years at Lakewood Fire District 2 in south Pierce County, Washington. Gary is actively involved locally and nationally as well as internationally. Chief Aleshire served as the Western Division President of the International Association of Fire Chiefs, and was a board member for over a decade. Gary continues to serve as a peer assessor team leader for the Center for Public Safety Excellence international accreditation process. Most recently, Gary successfully led the Souda Bay, Greece fire department through international accreditation status in excellence. Gary has also serves as an agency mentor for the CPSE's accreditation program project.

Chief Aleshire developed and implemented an organizational performance program for the fire service applying current theory and methodologies. In addition, Gary has developed and presented leadership programs to realign the culture and organizational delivery of public safety programs resulting from recent mergers or contracted services between multiple fire departments. These concepts aided in the successful consolidation of multiple fire jurisdictions to attain effectiveness and efficiencies across public safety programs.

Gary has also authored and presents his philosophy on "Success and Succession." This concept introduces and leads organizations why and how to support and believe in internal human capital for the long-term return on investment. These concepts blend traditional fire and business theory to fit the next generation of organizational service and excellence. Through the application of these ideals, Chief Aleshire was successful in maintaining a highly functional and respected relationship between labor/management representatives.

Gary is currently contributing as a subject matter expert and technical writer for a national company providing public safety policy and procedure programs. In addition, Gary continues to research and develop new concepts specific to integration of compensable service models leading to innovative pathway management of health care delivery through bridging out-of-hospital response with home health care.

Michael Anderson was a Firefighter/Paramedic for nine years and an Emergency Medical Technician for private ambulance for twenty-three years. He currently maintains his Emergency Medical Technician Certification, and is a court approved medical expert witness for emergency medical services incidents.

Michael is currently a Licensed Private Investigator and Paralegal. He has his own private practice: Anderson Investigations, LLC. Michael handles all types of cases, but specializes in civil litigation and family law. Michael is certified as a crime scene investigator, medico-legal death investigator and a written statement analyst.

Michael is a guest speaker at the private investigation course at the University of Washington on surveillance. He teaches at Washington State legal investigators conferences on "How to testify in court," and teaches a class on Washington Law, "When it's legal to shoot someone in self-defense."

Eddie Buchanan began his fire service career in 1982. He is a division chief with Hanover Fire & EMS in Richmond, Virginia. He is a past-president of the International Society of Fire Service Instructors, and serves on the advisory board for "Fire Engineering Magazine" and FDIC. He is the author of the Volunteer Training Officers Handbook, and serves on the Technical Committee for Fire Services Training for the NFPA. He is the 2015 recipient of the George D. Post, Instructor of the Year award from the ISFSI and FDIC. He has a bachelor's degree in Human Resource Management from the University of Richmond, and an associate's degree in Fire Science.

Angela Hughes began her experience with the career Fire Service in 1989 as a Paramedic with the Baltimore City Fire Department. She was hired by Baltimore County in 1992, and functioned as a Paramedic, Preceptor/Coach, Firefighter, Fire Marshal and Lieutenant. Hughes currently serves as a Captain assigned to the Chase station. As the co-founded of the Baltimore County Women in the Fire Service, she continues to mentor women and currently serves as the President of the International Association of Women in Fire and Emergency Services. Her Committee work includes the USFA Severity of House Fires, FEMA grant reviews, VCOS Diversity and Inclusion, National Fallen Firefighters Tampa 2, NFFF

Suicide Symposium and most recently NFPA Needs Assessment Summit. Captain Hughes has been published in Fire Engineering and has spoken several fire service venues.

Matthew Krueger has prior experience in both law enforcement and information security. He spent the last 9 years as the Lead Security Analyst at Digital Securus, where he has performed security and vulnerability assessments, developed policies, performed investigations, gathered localized intelligence on targets, as well as reconstructed evidentiary timelines from cellular and GPS data. He is heavily involved in the cyber counter-intelligence community as part of efforts to protect national critical infrastructure and multinational, US based businesses against advanced cyber-threats, and has been actively developing custom applications and detection processes for the purposes of Advanced Persistent Threat (APT) identification, analysis and reporting.

Introduction

This book is designed to address the unique challenges facing firefighters and emergency medical technicians (EMT) responding to individuals manifesting emotional disturbance, be it a symptom of mental illness, substance abuse, physical injury or psychological trauma. Our goal is to increase first responder and patient safety through specific strategies to quickly recognize and de-escalate threatening or aggressive patients' behavior(s).

The behaviors of mentally ill individuals can present as strange, even incomprehensible. What we do not understand seems hard to predict, leading us, at times, to perceive such individuals as dangerous, even when they are not. Through understanding such behaviors, you will become more skillful in assessing if a patient is truly dangerous, and in many situations, you will have the ability to calm them as well. You will often find that your presence alone prevents a situation from escalating, with patients complying with directives willingly, some even anxious to meet your approval or gain your respect.

Verbal de-escalation skills are on a continuum, with coaxing and reassuring the reluctant patient on one end, to verbal de-escalation and verbal control of paranoid, hyper-agitated or aggressive patients in the middle, and in some cases, physical restraint or self-defense against the truly violent. It is the hope of the authors, whose professional experience encompasses well over sixty years of face-to-face encounters with mentally ill and emotionally disturbed individuals, that this book will be invaluable in readying both newer first responders and experienced veterans for such encounters.

This book is about safety, first and foremost, but this subject goes far beyond managing to survive a shift uninjured. In addition to the threat of violence, firefighters and EMTs routinely face serious job-related pressure. Dealing with bizarre, profoundly distressed, mentally disordered patients can exponentially add to the rigors of the job. If first responders have confidence that they know the best way to communicate with these most confusing and sometimes dangerous patients, their very stressful job will become less so, and therefore, safer in the bargain.

We do not expect that all the information in this book will be new. You will have learned a lot of it, either in previous training or in the school of hard knocks. One service this book can provide is to confirm knowledge you already have. Sometimes you know something, but 'don't know you know.' When you bring such a skill to consciousness—one major purpose of this book—it will become part of your delivery system rather than something you almost accidentally come up with on those days you are 'dialed in.'

This book is part of a series of guidebooks for people who must face aggressive individuals. Other books in this series are specific to those who work as 9-1-1 call-takers and dispatchers, police officers, correctional officers, probation/parole officers, security professionals, inpatient units in hospitals, and social services personnel. There is also a separate version for families who live with mentally ill family members. Please refer to the website **www.edgework.info** for more information concerning both bound and ePub versions of all of these books.

The broad range of professionals who are discussed in this text

In some jurisdictions, firefighters are also emergency medical technicians (EMT). In other jurisdictions (the Midwest and East Coast of America, for example), they are two separate functions, and Emergency Medical Services (EMS) will arrive on scene separately in an ambulance. A majority of the fire service in this country is provided by volunteer firefighters, who face the same situations as the career firefighters. Among firefighters and emergency medical services are people with a wide range of medical training. These individuals are often called as a group 'first responders' regardless of their titles, training or certification—however, police officers and sheriff's deputies also referred to as first responders in many areas. To avoid any confusion, we will generally refer to "firefighters and EMTs" when referring to those who respond to emergency medical situations in the community.

SECTION I

Core Requirements For
De-escalation And Control Of
Agitated, Aggressive or
Mentally Ill Patients

CHAPTER 1

The Essentials

Firefighters and Emergency Medical Technicians (EMT) are the nation's first responders to many types of incidents: suppressing fires, rescuing individuals in car accidents, as well as medical aid calls concerning everything from lacerations, fractures and general illness to cardiac arrest. Newer first responder delivery models, under such names as a Community Paramedic system, address the needs of the chronically ill by directing their care to mental health or home health care agencies, placing these patients in a direct care program with the most appropriate providers.

Firefighters and EMTs are often called to assist patients in their communities because there is no one else to call. Not all of them are grateful, or even aware that we are there to help. We see many patients suffering from stress, intoxication, or just a bad attitude who violently attack firefighters or EMTs. Families of mentally ill individuals frequently call the fire department for assistance when their loved one needs to be transported to a medical facility, but all too often, those patients do not desire to go to the hospital and violently resist those efforts.

Firefighters and EMTs are injured every day on the job from all types of causes, including motor vehicle accidents, fires, cardiac events, building collapses as well as being attacked by our patients. Some studies indicate that about one third of firefighters and EMTs have been attacked by their patients: some with fists, knives, guns and other weapons. Hard statistics are hard to come by, as many first responders do not report such incidents unless they are medically treated for the injury. With over 1,400,000 firefighters and about 891,000 paramedics and EMTs in the United States, hundreds of thousands of first responders have surely been victims of assault.[1]

In the best of circumstances, firefighters and EMTs will be informed by emergency dispatch of potential danger before they arrive at a call. For example, the dispatcher reports a request for assistance in transporting a patient who has been off medications and is 'acting crazy,' or violently lashing out against family or caregivers. Police are usually dispatched as well, and strive to make the scene and patient secure before firefighters and EMTs contact the patient. However, in other occasions, there is no report of potential violence, and firefighters and EMTs walk into a scene that appears to be calm, but rapidly escalates into a violent attack. In rural areas with sparse law enforcement coverage, firefighters and EMTs may arrive at a scene before law enforcement. Different situations require different responses: sometimes, the first responders should defend themselves and exit the scene; in other situations, they should attempt to subdue the attacker to prevent harm to the patient and others; and in other times, they will make an attempt to 'talk the patient down' with some carefully crafted words and body language. The most important issue is to prevent harm to the first responders, other bystanders and the patient.

Although this book centers on verbal de-escalation skills, we must start at a more basic level, because the contributing causes of many critical incidents can be attributed to a lack of attention to basic safety precautions. This must begin *before* you start your workday. If your mind is unfocused, your ability to notice early warnings signs of potentially dangerous situations will be impaired. For example, fire fighters and EMTs cannot allow personal or familial issues to intrude upon their ability to focus on the job at hand.

The development of a general culture of safety is based upon the following three fundamental assumptions:
1. Being pro-active about safety issues must be a primary concern of your entire crew: managers, supervisors, first responders and support staff.
2. There needs to be consistency and a common understanding in the application of safety procedures and emergency protocols at all levels of the institution.
3. Adequate crew safety preparedness and situational awareness is not a once-and-done training event: ongoing communication is required between all levels, and a regular review of safety protocols, operational policies, crisis response processes, and ongoing training for all crew is crucial.

What Do We Mean by Mental Illness in the Context of De-Escalation?

What is a mental illness anyway? Is it any odd or eccentric behavior, or should we confine the term to more serious disturbances of behavior and thought? It sometimes seems that we lump together mental phenomena that are as disparate as the distinction between a common cold and lung cancer. Yes, both may make breathing difficult, but they are different, by orders of magnitude.

There should be no expectation that firefighters and EMTs diagnose what mental illness a patient may be suffering from, even in the most general way. This book focuses on behavior, not on specific mental health diagnoses. Nonetheless, if someone behaves in a way that makes it difficult to communicate with them, or even more problematically, enacts disruptive behaviors, then you should be prepared with several skills, among these are the following:
- The ability to recognize the behavior as showing a pattern.
- The knowledge of best practice communication strategies to respond to a person who is displaying such a pattern of behavior, whatever the cause may be.

Not everyone who needs to be calmed or de-escalated is aggressive. However, those who display unusual or eccentric patterns of behavior are more difficult to communicate with, and when the ability of people to communicate breaks down, the risk of aggression increases.

> ### Figure 1.1 Deal with the behavior, not the cause
>
> It is irrelevant whether a patient' behavior is driven by mental illness, drug intoxication, organic factors or just having a really bad day, until their behavior is under control. The general practice of the first responder is to mitigate the situation. Diagnosis comes later as the individual reaches a treating medical facility. When describing the patient's medical condition to a treating provider, it is best to describe the condition of the patient you found them in, and then describe their behavior. First responders are generally not trained in the diagnosis of mental illnesses, but they can describe behavior, what the patient (or family) tells them and the patient's response to field treatment. This is also the best course of action when documenting the interaction on your medical incident report form.

The reasons that drive a patient to violence are irrelevant until after the assault has been stopped. Aggressive behaviors, however, do not emerge in a vacuum. Without understanding what provoked or elicited the urge to be violent in the first place—anguish, frustration, confusion, boredom, fear, delight in terrorizing others, a drive to dominate or escape, to name only a few examples—we will never be able to circumvent the violence before it occurs.

Finally, unless we are aware if and when we are part of the problem—that our behavior or demeanor may have triggered the aggression in the patient—we will never be able to establish safety on scene.

Other Basic Requirements

1. **Follow standard procedures.** There MUST be standardized protocols for dealing with potentially or actually aggressive patients, as well as those who are mentally ill. It is true that one sometimes has to make an exception and go outside the rules, but you must understand that, in doing so, you are taking personal rather than institutional responsibility for your action. It may be the right thing to do, but you will have to prove it—not only by positive results, but also by your explanation. In any event, this must be the most unusual of occasions.

2. **Adaptability.** Notwithstanding the necessity for standardized procedures, firefighters and EMTs must also be flexible and creative. Standardization must never become inflexible and dogmatic, but rather, adaptable to the changes routinely occurring in a fluid, ever-changing environment.

3. **Solid boundaries.**
   - Your agency must be known as one where all staff members are vigilant in maintaining ethical and moral relationships in interactions with patients.
   - Everyone must ensure that interactions among your crew are professional—no one in your crew will act in any way among themselves that will negatively affect the care of patients, or compromise safety among your crew.

4. **Integrity.** Establishing safety for yourselves and your patients can only can occur when you offer the best of you to your profession. Without this, all the de-escalation methods in the world are just empty words.

5. **Empathy**. Empathy does not mean to 'feel sorry for someone.' That is sympathy. Empathy is the ability to 'track' another person—to get a sense of what they are feeling or experiencing from the sound of their voice, their facial expressions, and body language. The best emergency responders have an ability to get a 'felt sense' that something is wrong from the slightest of clues.

6. **Intuition**. This is the ability to become aware of small changes in people's tone of voice and pattern of speech as well as the surrounding environment such as crowds, neighborhood, and background noises that indicate that something else is happening beyond what is said. This can also be termed *situational awareness*. (Section II)

Training

As part of their initial and continuing education, first responders must be trained to recognized mental or behavioral health emergencies, and how to approach a patient with a mental illness or other behavioral disorder. For example, the Basic Emergency Medical Technician (EMT-B) curriculum has a brief chapter on Behavioral Emergencies that states: *"Develops the student's awareness of behavioral emergencies and the management of the disturbed patient. Restraining the combative patient will also be taught in this lesson."*[2] Subsequent to the basic EMT training for behavioral health issues, there are a number of resources where an EMT, Paramedic or other first responder can obtain advanced training relevant to their provision of emergency care for those with behavioral health issues. Given increasing numbers of individuals who are presenting with behavioral health emergencies, EMTs and Paramedics should incorporate behavioral training as part of their continuing medical education (CME) training requirements.

Cross-System Information Sharing

Information must be shared among all those concerned with a dangerous or at-risk mentally ill patient. This should include everyone from hospital staff, a mental health or substance abuse treatment agency, and/or local emergency first responders. All information that is associated with potential danger must be shared, not only for ethical reasons, but because it is the best way for everyone to remain safe. You will get feedback that you hadn't thought of, and furthermore, people will be prepared to help you.

Information sharing is not only an interagency question. Make sure all firefighters and EMTs within your department are aware of changes in behavior or verbalizations by any person of concern. Remember, although you may see the same people over and over again, they don't always act the same! All too often, someone is left out of the loop. The permutations are endless, but the consequences are dire. If all members of an organization aren't aware of dangerous elements within their perimeter, someone is very likely going to be hurt. For those reasons, use all available media to ensure that everyone has all necessary information within the confines of HIPAA.[3] Among the most problematic patients are so-called 'frequent flyers,' some of whom present a continual danger to the first responders. Such individuals require a measured and well-calculated response with sufficient staff and resources—without information sharing, this is not possible.

Past History Is Data—Not a Prediction

Let us imagine Ms. Smith, who chronically complains of shortness of breath, a medical condition. Her medical history would indicate she might have asthma or COPD. The treatment for her condition would be the same for each responder. For a person with a mental illness or behavioral health issues, however, each contact must be treated as a first time encounter, albeit referencing any information or experiences acquired in previous incidents. There is no assurance that you will be safe just because you've previously dealt with an individual in an effective way, or because previous reports describe a pattern. This doesn't mean previous success can't be repeated—however, persons suffering with mental illness can be extremely unpredictable. First responders must not become complacent. We have had several tragic incidents over the last decade where seasoned firefighters and EMTs were killed by a mentally ill patient, someone with whom the first responders had previously had many safe contacts.

Respect Is a Matter of Safety

Some mentally ill individuals have numerous contacts with firefighters and EMT, sometimes many times a week. Keep in mind they weren't always repeat customers. There was a first time. Their first encounter with a firefighter or EMT can often establish a positive or negative pattern for future encounters. Proper interaction is based on human respect, something accomplished through an air of quiet confidence and genuine interest in the other person, not through challenge or trying to appear tough.

We've each been sent on-scene with certain firefighters or EMT, and think, "Oh, this is going to go badly." There are, unfortunately, firefighters or EMT who make fun of someone or jack them up to the point that someone will have to go hands on with them. This should never be condoned by either first responders, or tolerated by the agency or medical authority. If a patient believes they're being demeaned or abused, they may remember that event and seek revenge in the future on yours or a different crew. All too frequently, they target all those whom they perceive associated with the abuser, seeing a uniform, rather than a specific individual who harmed them. It may be subsequent first responders, utterly unaware of the previous incident, who suffers the consequences if firefighters or EMT make fun of or otherwise demean a patient. Respect could be termed, 'banking for future' encounters with a patient.

Lesson #1 – Respect saves lives.

Figure 1.2 One author's experience—'banking for the future'

I once worked with a young man who had severe bipolar disorder. When on his medications, he was, for all intents and purposes, normal—a friendly, bright, and articulate guy. During the six months I saw him, we simply had friendly conversations and enjoyed each other's company. Approximately one year later, I was asked by another mental health agency to do a welfare check on him. I went to his apartment alone, and spoke with him a few minutes. Off his meds, he was irrational and psychotic. Sensing danger, I quickly left. He subsequently was detained for involuntary treatment, assaulting a number of police in the process. He was hospitalized over half a year. Sometime after his release, I ran into him in the street, once again on his medications and apparently doing well. He was overjoyed to see me, far more so than I thought the situation warranted. When I asked him why, he said, "I was afraid that you were dead. I remember you coming to my apartment, and I decided to kill you. I was just about to make my move when a voice went off in my head that said, 'You can't kill him, he's your friend.' I was arguing with the voice, because I couldn't remember what a friend was, but the voice said it was against the rules to kill friends. Then you were gone. For nine months, I've been hoping you left my apartment, but I couldn't remember. I've been afraid that I actually killed you, and buried you some place. I'm so glad to see you!!!"

Keeping Records as it Pertains to Violence

All EMS responses must generate a patient care report that records the pertinent medical information and treatment of the patient, either handwritten documents or electronic medical records. These forms are designed to record violent incidents and threats, and pass on information to other health care practitioners. They can also incorporate witness statements as part of medical information. These documents, created real-time, can assist the provider or their agency against legal challenges brought by the patient for allegations of excessive restraint, treatment protocols used to treat the patient and other pertinent information indicating appropriate care for this individual. When shared, this information helps all parties reduce further dangerous situations and provide documentation for future use, especially when reviewing your response to behaviorally ill patients. The medical record offers specific information, such as: the patient seems agitated and does not follow commands; was combative and speaking incoherently; threatened to harm herself by taking pills; indicated they were going to kill the responders.

If your department is utilizing electronic medical records, there should be a pop-up screen if you are responding to or have responded to a patient with a behavioral health history, and especially if there was a violent interaction with the first responders. Many times the responding apparatus (aid car, medic unit or fire engine) will have mobile data terminals (MDT) or other similar equipment that can contain this important patient information. Your dispatch center will often have a history file on these patients and can relay that information to the responders either through the MDT or over the radio. The dispatch centers need to be aware that non-essential individuals (civilians) may overhear this information by way of radio scanners, so the medical information relayed to the first responders must be concise and accurate, and not contain protected patient information such as name, address and social security number.[4]

In the electronic medical record, you can easily find repeat or similar incidents that may have led a person to be aggressive in the past. Through this, you may be able to discern patterns that help in predicting future incidents. Often, it is *only* when all the incidents are placed together that one is able to see a pattern to the aggression. EMS agencies participating in Quality Assurance programs will need to identify the aggression of the patient as part of the total patient care interaction with the providers. Continued awareness of this subject is essential to the safety of the providers.

For those agencies using hand written documentation, this search process, requiring cross-referencing is more difficult. Once solution is to have a specific section of charts where all notes concerning aggressive and violent incidents are copied and placed. Although this should be obvious, records should be printed or written in dark ink, and be immediately legible; unreadable handwriting is a form of malpractice, because data, unread, simply doesn't exist.

Figure 1.3 – An example of a pattern revealed after a record check

A young man, who frequently requires psychiatric aid, is always explosive in the second week of the month. After this is noticed, an investigation reveals that this is several days after he is required to visit his mother, who is court-ordered to have supervised visits. The visitation supervisor, a relative, frequently leaves the room to give them some "time alone," contrary to the court order, and he is subject to emotional abuse during these periods.

Lesson #2 – Records Save Lives

Threat Assessment for Firefighters and EMTs—After Action Review

In any aggressive and/or violent incident, it is essential to learn more about the patterns of behavior that might have preceded the patient's aggression, as well as any actions on the part of your crew (and other first responders such as police or dispatch) that were either unhelpful or contributory towards the patient becoming violent. Essential questions in any After Action Review (AAR) should include:

- What were the circumstances that led to the aggressive encounter?
- What was the *first* sign that indicated that the situation was getting volatile or dangerous?
- Remember what the patient said and what they did just before the aggressive incident.
- People are generally able to control their verbal signals better than their non-verbal signals, so recall the patient's body language prior to the incident. Tension can also create a change in the quality of the voice such as rate of speech, pitch, and/or volume.

- Consider what you physically felt at each stage of the encounter. This may be the most important data you can recover. The sensations evoked within the context of an encounter with another person are physical expression of intuition (Chapter 7). When you next experience that same sensation, it is an early warning sign that a similar situation is developing.[5]
- What do you believe you should have done differently?
- What were the results of the AAR of the incident? What did you learn?
- It is possible to incorporate this 'learning experience' as a tactical plan for other first responders who may not have had such an encounter with this patient, both for general training when encountering analogous situations and to develop a specific plan to prefer for future contacts with *this* patient.

Lesson #3 – Institutional Knowledge Saves Lives

CHAPTER 2

Safety In The Field

The Basic Emergency Call Process

Calls for assistance usually arrive at a Public Agency Answering Point (PSAP) located in the police or sheriff's department, or a consolidated call center containing both police and fire dispatchers. The PSAP will occasionally be located at the fire department itself. Regardless where the information is received, the call-taker must obtain essential information to ensure safety of both first responders and the subject of the call. This is especially important where there is a patient who may be at risk of harming themselves or others, or presents a known threat towards first responders.[6] However, the dispatcher may not be able to acquire this information, and the first responder will walk into a dangerous situation unaware. Therefore, you must always develop (and communicate) an exit strategy any time you enter a potentially volatile scene—and *any* emergency situation is volatile.

It is incumbent upon first responders to focus on their own safety, any non-involved individuals such as family members or bystanders, and as best as that can be accomplished, that of the patient. In many cases, this requires the assistance of additional personnel or law enforcement officers. Some regions also include mental health professionals who act as first responders when requested by police or fire departments in mental health emergencies.

Dealing with individuals with behavioral health issues often takes a time to resolve, not infrequently requiring one or two hours in the field. These are situations where you cannot "treat, load, and go," as you can in a medical emergency, due to the resistance of the patient. Once the scene is stable, therefore, it is important to communicate with the patient in a non-threatening manner. Patience, therefore, is a virtue for first responders.

Nonetheless, there must be a treatment plan formulated as quickly as possible, generally with the assistance of medical control and the patient's practitioner. Not infrequently, this may also require the use of 'overwhelming force' (by police or firefighters and EMTs) to get the patient loaded in the back of the ambulance (or other vehicle), and transported to a medical facility. Overwhelming force includes physical interventions, where you have enough hands available to make the patient helpless, or chemical restraints (both of which will be discussed later in this book) as methods of getting the patient to the hospital.

Figure 2.1 Responder safety is more than what occurs in the field

'Responder safety' does not only refer to what happens between firefighters and EMTs and the patient while on-scene. What you do or don't do can compromise your safety in other ways. For example, if you leave a patient home and they harm themselves or others, or even take their own life, not only was the patient and/or other citizens harmed, you can be sued for abandonment or depraved indifference.

In addition, a first responder can incur damaging psychological consequences, not only as an after-effect of violence, but also as a result of guilt at the failure to adequately protect yourself, your crew or your patient.

During the transport time, it is important is the patient is restrained in a physical position that does not inhibit his or her ability to breathe. Prior to transporting, reposition the patient to ensure an open airway and assess that the patient is actually breathing.

Violent episodes during transport can easily be mitigated with medications, administered by paramedics or other qualified practitioners. This is only possible if you have properly restraint and positioned the patient (See Appendixes A-C)

Your responsibility for the care of this patient usually ends upon arrival at the hospital or other treating facility. At this point, it is important that the patient is handed off to a qualified hospital practitioner, most likely a receiving nurse. The first responder must relay the medical information to the receiving nurse or other designated medical professional, including what occurred in the field, medications (if administered), and if restrained, the reasons for the restraints. Remember, the behaviorally disturbed patient is just as dangerous to the hospital staff as they may have been to you. Finally, good documentation of the event is required; if possible, complete that documentation prior to leaving the medical facility, or soon thereafter, if you need to respond to another emergency.

Don't Let the Abnormal Become Normal

Because firefighters and EMT are always working in the field, they must always consider potential danger. If you are already aware that a location is dangerous, of course you should secure police back-up, whenever possible. Sometimes, however, the danger is only apparent once you are in the middle of it. Don't let complacency cause career changing injuries. Be alert to the clues that something is not right.

We can't underscore how important it is to take note of and share your gut sense (physical intuition) that something is not right or dangerous with fellow firefighters and EMTs and, in many situations, with professionals outside the law enforcement arena. Not only should you be consulting with other responders when you're concerned about a patient, but just as important, *consult when you should be concerned and aren't*. Some firefighters and EMTs become so familiar with medical or psychological pathology that the abnormal becomes normal. They no longer react in a natural way, tolerating or not even noticing covert aggression, or pre-assault indicators.

Consider those you see so often that you refer to them by first name or even a nickname. You can easily become complacent because you deal with this person so often ("Oh, I know that guy. He's all mouth."). Remember the adage, "There is nothing routine in work." Don't get so focused on accomplishing a task that you ignore or discount signs of danger. Your job requires you to get up-close-and-personal; even so, never forget how quickly and easily you can become a victim of violence.

Figure 2.2 Don't hand them a weapon

We've seen far too many firefighters and EMTs leaning over patients with 'sharps' (scissors, knives, etc) in a little holster on their belt or in their pockets, well within reach of the patient they are putting in restraints.

There are some in the firefighter/EMS industry calling for the ability of such first responders to actually carry weapons: handguns, stun guns or chemical defense weapons. As any police officer will tell you, this is a dangerous idea. One of the most important actions a police officer does if attacked or assaulted is to defend his or her weapons. They undergo extensive training in weapon-retention as well as deployment and use of weapons, neither of which is the primary duty of a firefighter or EMT. In general, assaults by patients are sudden and violent, and occur when you are primarily focused on rendering medical assistance, not like a police officer who goes into a scene anticipating and primarily prepared for the possibility of a violent attack. It is highly unlikely that you will have time to deploy any weapon system effectively, and it is more likely that whatever you are carrying will be used against you.

Lesson #4 – Stowing Potential Weapons Saves Lives

Before Going on a Response

Dispatch should have dangerous residences and individuals 'flagged,' whenever possible (Chapter 1). Calls regarding such a residence or individual should automatically activate police involvement and a warning of the potential dangers to firefighters and EMTs.

Approaching the Scene

As you approach the scene, you should be surveying your surroundings.
- You should look for escape routes, safe havens, and blind spots where you cannot see if someone is hiding.

- Listen for sounds of conflict both in the surrounding neighborhood and emanating from the scene.
- Look for people 'assessing' you. Distinguish between curiosity, hostility, and outright menace.

DO NOT talk yourself out of any feelings of trespass or danger. Your GUT feelings play an important role in your safety. If the situation seems unsafe, then do not continue to the patient's location without police!

At the Scene

1. Knock on the door or ring the doorbell with your safety in mind.
   - Whenever possible, we advise that you stand away from the center of the door as the unstable patient may slam it into you, or even shoot a firearm through the door.
   - Check the hinges to see if it opens outward or inward. If the door opens outwards (toward you), step back and stand on the hinge side of the door, well back, so it is not slammed into you.
   - If it opens inwards (away from you), step back and stand on the handle side so that if they intend to yank open the door and strike at you, you will not immediately be in line of the blow.
   - If the landing or porch is narrow and there is not room for that, stand well back from the door, after you knock.
   - If you must stand at the top of some stairs, hold onto something with one hand so that, were you suddenly pushed, you would have a chance of protecting yourself from a dangerous fall.
   - Stop screen doors with a foot to keep dogs from lunging out at you.

2. Do not approach the scene with your arms full. We have a tendency to carry too much medical equipment to these types of calls. Most of the equipment is not necessary, and you must be in a position to defend yourself. At least one arm should be free.

3. When you enter the scene, be aware of doors that can lock behind you essentially trapping you with your aggressor. You can use a wedge or other blocking devices, or duct tape over the door latch to keep the door open for a safe exit from the room or home.

4. Do not lose focus on your patient and be distracted by other individuals in the room. You can perform a quick survey from the doorway to see potential threats, including other angry individuals, weapons or even dogs. (This includes even the smallest dog—they may not be able to reach higher than your ankle, but they can still leave a nasty laceration, sometimes followed by an even more nasty infection).

5. As described above in the section on assessing the environment, survey the room for anything out of place. Whenever possible, try to also assess other rooms in the house, not only for people or objects that might be dangerous, but in general, an understanding of a patient's living environment can be very telling.

Figure 2.3 Authors' examples of surveying for safety:

I once entered the house of an elderly woman suffering from paranoia and dementia. In a quick survey of the room, I saw two dark items uncharacteristically protruding from a beaded curtain. Upon checking, I realized that she had thrust two large butcher knives in the frame of the window. Her plan was that if some unwanted person entered her home (and here I was!), she would back up to the window, and yanking out the knives, disembowel the invader. Had I not spotted the knives and gotten to them first, I might not be writing these lines now.

In another call, the owner had two Doberman pinschers, which were barking and lunging at us through the door. We asked the owner to put the dogs into a bedroom and close the door. He did what we asked, and we entered the home. Just to be safe, however, we called for police and animal control. After a brief time, the patient got unhappy with us, becoming increasingly agitated. He made a beeline to the bedroom door, intending to set the dogs free. We ran out of the house, leaving our equipment behind, and jumped into the aid car. The dogs proceeded to attack the aid car, and chewed or tore off the mirrors and emergency lighting, then attacked the tires, before being subdued by the police and animal-control officer. We then re-entered the home with a police escort. The patient was arrested for assault on a public safety officer, was transported in the back of our now chewed-up aid car to the hospital, and then transferred to jail after medical treatment.

Lesson #5 – Knowing What's Around You Saves Lives

Field or Situational Awareness

You must be conscious of what a potential aggressor is doing, and what it probably means. Remain conscious of:

- **Where are your escape routes?** Is something blocking your way out?
- Are there any **obstacles**, sharp corners or other hazards that you need to avoid?
- **Are there any weapons** around that can be used against you, or in the worst case, that you can pick up in your own defense?
- **Is the person's aggressiveness escalating?** If so, what is the proximate cause of their escalation, and what mode of aggression are they moving into? (See the latter sections of this book).
- Does their threat display have a secondary purpose? Do they have **allies** who are waiting for you to get off-guard, at which point they will join in the attack?
- What are *your* non-verbal behaviors? **Are you getting mad too?** If so, it is best to disengage; if not, you will merely get very angry together, and the situation could become explosive.
- **Where is your 'team?'** Where are the police? Are other firefighters and EMTs aware of the danger, and what are they doing to help control the scene?

CHAPTER 3

Safety In The
Emergency Room

Avoiding Catastrophe in the ER. Helping Others to Help the Patient

Emergency rooms are a special consideration when considering staff and patient safety. This is not because there is a special patient population that visits the emergency room—they are the same individuals you see, even the same individuals you have just transported to the ER. The medical practitioners in emergency rooms, if confronted by an aggressive patient, must use the same strategies of verbal de-escalation and control that they would use in any another setting.[7] The patient with behavioral issues must be secured to prevent self-harm or harm to the staff or to other waiting patients, because someone can easily be hurt during the transition from your care to theirs.

Do not Compromise Your Safety

Do not enter a situation that, by definition, puts you in danger. Ask, request, and then demand, if necessary, that emergency room personnel assist you in making the situation safe enough for you to do your job. This can include direct intervention with the patient, administering chemical restraint, placing the patient into a restrictive garment or moving them to a safe or holding room with a trained attendant. Emergency room staff must never leave such patients unobserved

The Dangers

In many states, law mandates or convenience dictates that patients in psychiatric emergencies are taken to the nearest emergency room, whether or not that facility is equipped for psychiatric emergencies in general, and even worse, whether or not it is ready to manage assaultive individuals. The problems include:

1. **No safe place for the patient to be**. Many hospitals do not have a seclusion room where the patient can both rest safety and be secured. Quite frequently, the patient is left in a room full of weapons of opportunity—sharps, syringes, and any number of items that can be used as bludgeoning instruments or projectile weapons. With startling frequency, suicidal patients are left unattended with full access to a huge variety of items: medication and cutting instruments that they can—and occasionally do—use to attempt suicide. In addition to the potential for patients to attempt suicide, there is also the risk that they may harm staff or other patients.

2. **Understaffed for emergencies**. Many smaller emergency rooms are understaffed at night. There are not sufficient individuals at smaller hospitals to assist in, for example, restraint procedures if they are needed. Of even greater concern, many hospitals give their staff no training whatsoever in this area. When transporting a patient to this type of facility it is recommended that your

crew remain with the patient until there is sufficient staff assembled to transfer this patient to the control of the hospital.

3. **No security staff or too few in numbers**. Many smaller hospitals do not have any security personnel, or only one on duty; you may find yourself becoming defacto security staff.

4. **Poorly trained security staff**. Many hospitals are staffed by security guards that have no training whatsoever in communication with mentally ill or intoxicated individuals.[8] Many have little to no training in effective physical restraint appropriate to medical or psychiatric emergencies. The interventions of such undertrained or untrained security guards have, on occasion, exacerbated a situation rather than calming it down.

5. **Disempowered security staff**. We are aware of a number of major hospitals that have a rather large security force. However, they are forbidden to physically intervene with disruptive patients, and when called, are required merely to stand and observe. Reportedly, such hospitals are concerned about liability issues. Nurses and EMTs end up fighting with patients, while security staff watches nearby. The end result is that the hospital has, in essence, no functioning security staff, merely uniformed "observers." You and hospital staff end up on your own.

6. **An interpretation of patient rights against illegal search and seizure puts staff at risk**. Many hospitals, however staffed, will not, or cannot search patients for weapons or drugs. There have been many incidents of patients using either of these items as a weapon against themselves or others. In fact, you can search the patient while conducting your hands-on medical examination. You can also ask the patient if they have any weapons or exposed needles. However, what do you do with this information? You need to know what to do once a patient admits having a weapon. You need to know, both legally and operationally, how you can secure a weapon that the patient is willing to hand over, or that you simply discover in their clothes. As this can vary in different areas, request legal advice from your agency's attorney and request practical instruction from local law enforcement.

7. **In many states, due to inadequate beds in both the mental health and drug/alcohol treatments systems, many involuntarily committed patients are literally being 'boarded' in the emergency rooms for an entire 72-hour hold.** Such patients are not getting the clinical treatment they need. Not surprisingly, they present with severe management problems in an already over-stressed setting. In some states, there are new regulations either passed or pending to prevent boarding of patients. You must clearly understand the 'boarding legislation' in your state so that you are not in violation of the law, much less compromising patient care.

8. **Inadequate assessment**. Particularly with intoxicated or otherwise difficult-to-manage individuals, there is frequently an inadequate risk assessment. Ironically, patients who are demanding, obnoxious or otherwise hard to communicate with, may receive less assessment than more. A proper risk assessment should include a history of violence and suicide. Particularly with long-term patients in the 'system,' this information should be immediately accessible to emergency personnel—confidentiality laws being suspended in emergent situations. Procedures need to be in-place through which hospital and/or mental health personnel execute a 'one-touch' or 'one-call' access to information regarding violent history.

9. **Inadequate resources.** When an individual does not meet criteria for what should be the least restrictive alternative, both mental health and hospital personnel have few alternative referrals. This leads to patient and family outrage, and/or the crisis continuing to fulminate until the patient truly presents an unmanageable risk. Examples include:

   - <u>Detox</u> – Many detox facilities refuse to take dual diagnosis patients, particularly when their mental health issues, whatever the etiology, are severe. Although allegedly secure settings, many detox units do not have locked units, and the staff have little training or skill in dealing with mental health issues.[9] With no other option, these patients are taken by default to ER. Often with a criminal or anti-social history, they present severe risks to both staff and patients, particularly because they are not receiving treatment appropriate to their condition.

   - <u>No voluntary options</u> – a patient in a psychiatric emergency requests hospitalization, but may not be considered suitable for a voluntary unit, for any one of a number of reasons (previous acts of violence, non-compliance with rules, insisting on smoking in a no-smoking facility, sexualized behaviors, to name only a few). They are then 'cut loose,' even though they are in an emergent psychiatric state. Ironically, because they requested hospitalization, many jurisdictions will not place them in a more secure, 'involuntary' unit, even though that would properly assure both their own and public safety.

Figure 3 Lifesaving Points in Section I

Lesson #1 – Respect Saves Lives.

Lesson #2 – Records Save Lives

Lesson #3 – Institutional Knowledge Saves Lives

Lesson #4 – Stowing Potential Weapons Saves Lives

Lesson #5 – Knowing What's Around You Saves Lives

SECTION II

Centering: Standing With
Strength And Grace
In Crisis Situations

CHAPTER 4

Introduction To Centering

Dealing with patients who are mentally ill, drug dependent, victims of traumatic events, or struggling with developmental disabilities, brain injuries or personality disorders is an honorable calling. You will be in a position to help some of the most unfortunate members of society. Some will be extremely thankful; however, some may also be extremely dangerous.

Although your field and possible transport time with the patient is relatively short, the interaction can be very intense. Being confused, distracted, or intimidated by a mentally ill patient can easily lead to poor decision-making. Even more troubling is to realize that your reactions to such people sometimes make things worse. Even when you don't express your negative feelings, internalizing them can lead to 'burnout,' a kind of 'slow-motion post traumatic stress disorder.' Burnout can cause you to not pay attention at moments when awareness is most necessary

Stress Is a Safety Issue

This is surely one of the most stressful jobs in the world. It is a different kind of stress from a war zone, where one tries to survive in the midst of enemy fire. Rather, the firefighter and the EMT, by choice, go into emergent situations, where assaults are not an everyday occurrence, but they can happen in an instant. It is a world of constant *potential* threat, and rare actual violence. Such high levels of stress can lead to impaired judgment, even substance abuse problems, as well as a myriad of stress-related medical or personal issues. Stress can fuel cynicism or anxiety, as well as eliciting feelings of contempt towards certain types of individuals. When ingratitude or even hatred is the reward for caring, even heroic actions, the firefighter or EMT may become embittered. To risk so much and sometimes receive so little in return can affect one's home life, even leading to divorce or dysfunctional relationships with one's significant other or children.

There are ways to mitigate stress for crew who are overwhelmed. These include structured peer support programs, and employee assistance programs (EAP). There is no doubt that good leadership has a profound effect on staff morale and institutional safety. Good leadership supports a culture of safety, dignity, respect, and accountability. Supervisor or peer assistance in identifying crew members who are struggling is invaluable in getting them the help they require. Sometimes, however, nothing from 'outside' can help. Stress must be addressed from within, something we will also address in this section.

The strategies in the following chapters revolve around maintaining self-control. This is the ability to adapt to circumstances in a fluid and purposeful way. This attitude is essential to crisis situations. Emotionally disturbed patients are far more likely to comply with our directives when we are centered and in control.

Figure 4.1 Centering—it's all about tactics

We had a small dilemma with this section. Given that it includes tactical breathing methods, and an awareness of triggers that an aggressor could use to set you off-balance, we were concerned that some readers might interpret this as 'touchy-feely' stuff. It's not.

What it comes down to is this: all the tactics in this book are dependent on being centered. You can say all the right things, but if you aren't 'lined up right,' they will be of no use.

The more control you have over 'you,' the more certain you will say and do the right thing. This is true whether it involves walking down a hallway with flames behind the walls, or dealing with an aggressive patient who is burning with rage in front of your eyes.

Lesson #6 – Centering Saves Lives

CHAPTER 5

Peer Support Is A Survival Tactic

Feeling helpless or shamed after experiencing a physical or emotional attack is one of the worst experiences of one's life. This is particularly true on our jobs, because our professional pride is also attacked. When placed in fear of losing our life or well-being, we can feel profoundly isolated. We replay the incident in an incessant loop, over and over. This sense of isolation and helplessness gets far worse if there is no one with whom we can talk about what happened, and some of these incidents are so ugly or appalling that we are reluctant to discuss them with our spouses or other family members. To do so would be inviting violence or obscenity into our homes, and we don't wish to pass that kind of burden on to a loved one.

In such circumstances, you need *fair witnesses*, people, often fellow firefighters and EMTs, who know you, who respect you, and who are willing to hear you out. Such peer support can include strategizing sessions, (debriefings) or tactical review, but we (authors) must underscore that there are times that this is the last thing you need. The problem is not one of tactics—it is how the incident affected you. The presence of a fair witness informs you, often simply by being there, that you are still a part of the crew, and that your negative, even traumatic experience, is not unique to you, but something that any one of your teammates might experience. Sometimes the need for a fair witness surfaces during an after-action review. A firefighter or EMT may be 'stuck' on an error, or circumstances may lead them to either lose trust in themselves, in a teammate or in the system as a whole. Beyond corrective action, this is often the sign that peer support is needed.

> **Figure 5.1 Safety works both ways**
>
> To some of our readers, this chapter may seem far from a discussion on safety, but when we talk about someone "having our back," it doesn't only mean that they're with us while going through the door physically, but also when we see the tough or heartbreaking call, or there are problems off-duty. If we don't have an assurance that someone will be there when we return, it's a lot harder to go through the door in the first place.

Many organizations have begun to train their officers and firefighters to recognize stress in first responders after a traumatic call. Firefighters and EMTs often defuse the situation by talking things out on scene or soon afterwards. This process can sometimes be rowdy: full of teasing and rude jokes that may be startling to outsiders. This is not usually disrespectful—rather, it is a coping mechanism for people to deal with long term stress, punctuated by both danger and the witnessing of the terrible things that people do to themselves and others. Still, you must be careful. Both writers are aware of incidents where responders have been decompressing/joking and family members walk into the scene: this can be devastating for them. Secondly, given the nature of a team composed of a number of alpha males and females, this can sometimes become a competitive back-and-forth for 'shock value,' resulting in a de-sensitization and cynicism towards some patients, particularly individuals suffering from mental illness, drug abuse, or other disorders.

If stress-related problems are major or the affected first responders are not communicating, there may need to be a more formal response. Sometimes department chaplains can be an invaluable resource for individual crew members. Many agencies have incorporated a system of peer support, referred to by such terms as critical incident response teams (CIRT), critical emergency response teams (CERT), critical incident stress management (CISM), or critical incident stress debriefing (CISD). CISM members are fellow firefighters and EMTs who are trained to respond to critical events within the agency, and provide the affected firefighters and EMT with emotional support and assistance shortly after the event occurs. (NOTE: we will offer general principles here—there are different CISM models, and we are not, here, endorsing one over another).

A critical incident is an extraordinary event that forces firefighters and EMTs to face vulnerability and mortality during the course of their official duties. These incidents typically occur without warning and jeopardize one's physical safety or emotional well-being. Incidents such as being victimized in an assault can overwhelm one's stress capacity. A prompt and structured response can reduce the negative consequences of such incidents, and help restore the affected firefighters and EMTs equilibrium.

There are several steps team members may take in order to begin the healing process for affected first responders. It is imperative the CISM team members are trained and respected members of the organization. The interaction with the first responder should be in a quiet place without distractions. There should be open and honest discussions between the first responder and CISM member discussing the call, and the effects on the first responder and possibly their family. The department must have a CISM or Behavioral Health Policy, and have well trained members on staff. It may be well worth the effort to begin a Regional team, in order to have a broad base of trained responders and to assist in cost sharing among the department members.

5.2 Being 'voluntold'

Some people do not regain equilibrium through self-disclosure, particularly in group process. In this wise, mandatory CISM may be counter-productive for many. A range of options, centered around peer support, is best. Mandatory CISM, following a 'cookie' cutter' style, in which everyone is expected to heal the same way may be counter-productive, not only for the person who doesn't process trauma well in this manner, but also for others in the group who may be distracted by their disgruntled fellow firefighter or EMT.

At the same time, some individuals try to 'gut' things out alone, when they desperately need some help. Without a requirement from one's supervisor, such people may not get the help that they truly need.

Typically, the CISM member will contact the affected firefighters and EMT once a week for at least one month following the incident, and remain in contact with them until they're confident that the affected firefighters and EMTs physical and emotional needs have been addressed. If necessary, they will provide a referral to a professional counselor trained in the effects of trauma on first responders.[10]

Figure 5.3 The debate concerning documentation

CISM is used for a variety of professions besides fire fighters and Emergency Medical Services. Some CISM protocols recommend submitting a critical incident report to the administrative unit for the purpose of collecting information necessary to provide short-term and long-term assistance to the affected firefighter or EMT and to document activities, services, and progress.

Such record keeping can be problematic. Although this report should not to be used as an investigative tool, it can be. As an official record, it may also be subpoenaed in a lawsuit or other legal proceeding. Therefore, many CISM protocols recommend that nothing should be put in writing. This helps the affected firefighter or EMT feel like he/she can talk more freely. For firefighters and EMTs, the authors recommend that CISM teams take no notes. It should be noted that CISM and peer-support communication is 'privileged,' which protects the conversation from discovery by attorneys.

Written records should be confined to formal after-action, non-medical reviews. If the first responder needs to seek outside assistance through a referral or other mechanism, the mental health practitioner can contact the department and begin the process for time-off under the department's disability protocols. The practitioner will place the need for time-off in neutral terms, and not reveal the first responders actual medical condition. This will avoid a possible HIPAA violation. It is up to the firefighter or EMT to decide whether or not to give permission to the practitioner to share confidential information with certain members of their department (primarily Human Resources) to craft a successful 'treatment and return-to-work plan.'

Lesson #7 Peer Support Saves Lives

CHAPTER 6

It's Not Personal
Unless You Make It So

Firefighters and EMTs must take care to not personalize any disagreements or altercations with patients, no matter what the provocation. Unless you are in a struggle for your life, <u>you do not have to win</u>. Your goal is to establish peace so you can do your job—getting the patient to medical care. Negatively reacting to an aggressive patient, perhaps mentally ill, will cloud a firefighter or EMTs judgment, while distracting him/her from legitimate safety and medical concerns.

Beyond that, their attacks on you might *seem* personal, but that is only true if you make them so. If the attack is false, why take offense? On the other hand, if what the aggressor said is valid, then you're reacting in anger when someone tells you the truth. You knew it anyway, so what are you upset about?

- They call you fat? Well, you knew that already, didn't you?
- They called you a son of a bitch? You aren't, so why are you taking it personally?

Any attempt to 'get even,' is unacceptable to a professional. Your actions must be the result of unbiased decision-making based on the facts at hand. A move towards revenge is a manifestation of an attempt to assert dominance over the other as opposed to an attempt at establishing either safety or conflict resolution. When mentally ill patients push your buttons because of what they say or do, *it is an act of valor not to respond in kind.*

Obscenity and Verbal Violation

Some people use obscenity and other verbal violation to get you focused on what they're saying rather than what they're doing—such as closing the distance so they can attack you. Others may have had no initial intention to physically assault you—they were just spewing nasty slurs—but they suddenly realize that you, upset at what they just said, have lost focus and are open to attack. Still others suddenly perceive *in your response* to what they said that you have 'lost it,' and they 'attack you back first,' because they believe you're about to react. Others challenge you by trying to offend you or through trying to make you explain yourself. Provocative challenges are for the purpose of getting leverage on you.

No One Will Own Me

The verbal aggressor is trying to 'push your buttons,' often in an attempt to elicit an unprofessional or off-centered reaction. We are biologically organized to respond to danger through pattern-recognition that engenders a rapid reaction by the more primitive areas of the brain. A large object moving rapidly towards us, a sudden pain, or a violent grab initiates a cascade of responses—fight/flight/freeze/faint/

flinch—that are geared to keep us alive in the worst of circumstances. At lower levels of danger, particularly that presented by another human being, we're provoked into posturing—dominance/submission displays—that serve to maintain or enhance our position in a social structure.

The curse of being human, however, is that these survival responses are precipitated by any noxious stimuli, particularly those that shock or surprise us. When someone unexpectedly violates our sense of right and wrong or verbally assaults us, we automatically shift into those primitive responses, even when survival is not truly an issue. **When our buttons are pushed, we react as if we're threatened with bodily harm.**

Bracketing

Anything that puts you off-balance puts you at risk. It is essential, therefore, that you are aware of what your buttons are. Beyond self-awareness, however, use a technique called **bracketing** to make it harder, if not impossible, for others to even get to your buttons.

Not surprisingly, we are most likely to lose our temper—our flexibility, our edge and our strength— when we are blind-sided. Sudden emotional shock elicits the same responses in the nervous system as a physical attack. For example, if someone suddenly insults your race, religion, or gender, it is very likely that you will shift into a response using those parts of your brain that express raw emotions. The limbic system is not concerned about the truth, about negotiation, or how to make peace. Instead, it views the world as one at war, with the other person trying to destroy one's position of strength.

Here's a worksheet that can help you name and bracket your own hot buttons. (You can make a photo-copy to work on it separate from the book). Some example statements may include:
1. I can't stand it when someone attacks or demeans < >, because that's something I love and treasure.
2. I feel outraged when someone demeans < > because it is something I believe to be unquestionably right and good.
3. People get me defensive when they say or point out < >, because, to tell the truth, I hate it in myself or, it is a flaw....
4. When people say or do < >, I lose it because it's as if they're taking control of me, or disrespecting me.
5. They better not say < >. That's the one word I won't take from anyone.

Statement	Why Does this Get to Me?
EXAMPLE: When people say or do < >, I lose it because it's as if they're taking control of me, or disrespecting me.	

Taking Inventory

To keep others from knocking you off center, do the equivalent of checking your medical or fire equipment before going out into the field. **Every morning, upon waking, and maybe even a few times during the day, simply run an inventory, as if flipping through a set of cards, and call to mind each of your emotional triggers.** By waking your mind up to these vulnerabilities, you will not be caught off guard when someone tries to set you off. Without surprise, you will be far less likely to be involuntarily reactive.

Some people might believe this sort of inventory is either depressing or unnecessary, but that is no more realistic than regarding the requirement to check your mirrors before backing out of your driveway as an unfair burden. When (not 'if'), an aggressor or co-worker tries to push one of your buttons, you are internally prepared for it without being anxious about it. If you take inventory, you center yourself for another day, ready for the worst without it tearing you down. When your safety and that of your crew is on the line, this should not be considered a burden—it's the intelligent thing to do.

By the way: it would be great if this were a kind of self-therapy that would help you accept what you don't like about yourself. It's not. The purpose is for you to become aware enough of your triggers that when people launch any verbal attacks, you're prepared to deal with them, already balanced. The only thing that you will take personally is your own dignity.

You must establish a steady infallible core, both for yourself and for the people around you. You are obligated to the other members of your crew to refrain from escalating a situation, even when the patient pins you with some sudden insight or 'tell' that they read in you. You must present yourself as the embodiment of strength and calm, both for yourself and your crew, especially when your teammates are scared or otherwise off-balance.

CHAPTER 7

Training Your Intuition (Situational Awareness)
To Pick Up Danger

Developing Situational Awareness

Awareness of potential escape routes, likely weapons, and access to additional help should become a natural part of the firefighter and EMTs personal and professional life. This routine attentiveness is often referred to as 'situational awareness.' Some folks are naturally good at this and others are not. This section offers a method to teach firefighters and EMTs how to pick up danger on an intuitive level.

Enter a room or even stand near your ambulance or rig with a predator's mind and a predator's movements: slowly, gracefully, with calculation. Imagine that you are going to hurt the next person who comes into proximity. How would you cut off their escape routes? What could you use as a weapon? Where would you position yourself to attack? How could your victim best escape? Do the same thing, as best you can, recalling the behaviors of a psychotic or disorganized patient. Imagine a number of uniformed individuals suddenly appear, moving purposefully, but doing things you do not understand. How would you try to escape? What around you frightens you most? What enrages you most?

This technique, called 'shapeshifting,' can be enacted on an occasional basis, and can be a way to get insight into the minds of the people who may present a danger to you. Done over time, you will start to develop the ability to automatically scan any location to see if there is anything there which makes it a place of danger, as well as switching your mind on to picking up predatory or other dangerous behaviors on the part of others.

Intuition: That Small Voice to Which You Must Listen

Intuitions are sometimes vague, but they are often the *first* signs that one is in a dangerous situation. Don't keep them to yourself!

- Firefighters and EMTs, whether seasoned veterans or newer members of your crew, should never minimize their gut feelings and intuitions when exchanging information. Don't begin by stating "I know it's nothing, but…." In doing so, you may lead others to minimize the situation as well.
- Firefighters and EMTs should never be hesitant in speaking up even when they don't have 'hard evidence' to support their concern.
- Veteran firefighters and EMTs or senior staff members must not belittle other firefighters and EMTs' intuitions of danger. Even the most senior member of your crew has not experienced every possible contingency. Experience is not always the best teacher in these situations. It is important to not minimize your or your team's gut feelings about a call.

Figure 7.1 Example of lifesaving intuition

I just returned to the United States after spending a tour in Vietnam as a combat corpsman with the Marines. After discharge, I joined a fire department as a paramedic firefighter. One of the first calls I went on was a disturbed Vietnam veteran who expressed the desire to take his own life. Thinking I had some experience with military veterans, my partner and I called for police assistance and made entry into the home, calling out that we were with the fire department and were there to help. The individual's wife, who had called 9-1-1, met us at the door. I asked if the patient had any weapons, and she said that he did, but she had hid them. We proceeded carefully up the stairs to the bedroom where the patient was lying on the bed. I identified myself as a paramedic firefighter and former Marine Corpsman and he said, "Doc I am glad you are here to witness my death." He proceeds to roll over on the bed, pulled out a handgun and pointed it at his head. My gut instinct was to run, but my training and reaction was to disarm him. I yelled "GUN!" to my partner, and I jumped on the patient, wrestling the gun away from him. My partner joined the fray, and we subdued the patient, who proceeded to start crying. After the police arrived and restrained him, we transported him to the local hospital for treatment. He thanked me for stopping his suicide. He told me that he was trying to get help, but there were no resources available for military veterans. I thanked him for not shooting me, and he stated he would not have harmed a hair on my head because he was a Marine as well, and knew that his Corpsman would take care of him. In retrospect, my own intuition informed me of that fact, which is what I attribute my move towards the gun rather than retreating out of the room.

One other point: despite his wife's assurances, I entered the room, ready for anything and thus did not freeze. The best way to put it is that I was surprised—but not surprised—when he revealed the gun, and therefore, I was able to immediately act.

Authors' note: The reader should not mistake the action described above as our proscription for how to act every time a weapon appears. In most instances, of course the proper response should be immediate retreat. However, we chose this example deliberately to underscore that intuition sometimes demands exceptions to a rule or procedure—perhaps one is too close to retreat or perhaps one simply has an over-riding sense that a certain action is demanded, just as a firefighter, about to step on a floor in a burning building, stops, just as the floor collapses. Anyone who works emergencies knows that there are times when gut-sense must override standard operating procedures.

Lesson #8 – Intuition Saves Lives

Honing Intuition Through Awareness of Personal Spacing

Communicating with mentally ill people is most difficult when they're becoming agitated. Agitated people experience words, particularly a lot of them, as confusing, aggravating, and/or threatening. For all these reasons, keep whatever you say simple, using short sentences.

Beyond what you say, the agitated patient is paying more attention to other aspects of communication: muscular tension, the amount of physical space between you, the positioning of your hands, and the quality of your voice. As you evaluate the other person's potential for violence, they are doing the same.

The firefighter or EMT must take care to remain calm and prepare for the possibility of a physical confrontation, while simultaneously maintaining focus on verbally de- escalating the situation. **Most importantly, you should not feed the anger, particularly by losing your own temper.** Most people can't sustain anger for more than a couple of minutes, so if you can keep your composure, many patients will calm down on their own.

Lesson #9 – Being Cool Saves Lives

Learning pre-assault indicators, particularly 'body language,' is not enough. Although the **basic** emotions are expressed in definitive ways, irrespective of culture,[11] non-verbal behaviors can be idiosyncratic: not only do people often have their own ways of physically expressing their emotions, but they also have their own ways of interpreting (or misinterpreting) yours.

Firefighters and EMTs must hone their intuition to detect subtle warning signs that a dangerous situation is developing. The leading edge of intuition is a sense of personal space. This is not just a matter of feet and inches. How much space would you want if the person has a blade, or is twice your size and half your age?

Our attitude can also affect our sense of space. For example, the more relaxed you are in the company of someone you trust, the less personal space you require (something that manipulative aggressors try to take advantage of). When you are uncertain or suspicious of someone, you instinctively move to get more distance from them. If you are having a bad day, you need more space to tolerate anyone's proximity. You need to be familiar with your 'defensive space,' that which is necessary to provide time to react to an aggressive move by your patient. Complicating things for firefighters and EMTs is the fact that your professional responsibilities require you to be at intimate range, with your hands on their body, and yours, well within reach.

Lesson #10 – Awareness of interpersonal space saves lives

Figure 7.2 Two cautions concerning personal space
1. DON'T knowingly step inside someone's personal space, unless doing so helps you establish a clear tactical advantage, or is required to fulfill your professional responsibilities
2. DON'T accommodate anyone by allowing them to be too close to you, unless it is required to fulfill your professional responsibilities

You MUST be aware of and respond to the physical sensations of someone in your 'zone.' For example, with bystanders or family members, you set such a limit as "Sir, I very much wish to hear what you have to say, but you are standing too close. Move back and then we will continue to talk." This should be stated in a matter-of-fact tone, where you are assuring the person that in moving back, communication will be *improved*, rather than cut off.

By the way, it is not a 'failure,' if they get offended or belligerent when told to step back. Whatever reply you get will be excellent threat assessment information. You are dealing with very different individuals when one, told to step back, responds with profuse apologies compared to someone who smirks and says, "What's the matter, are you nervous around men?"

The Brain Wants to Survive

There are parts of the brain that are solely concerned with survival, that don't care about being polite, politically correct, or intellectualizing why someone is the way they are. These parts of the brain don't even use words. They perceive by recognizing significant patterns, and signal their recognition through physical sensations. The survival sections of the brain are fast—about half a second faster than the thinking brain. About to step on a squiggly shape on the ground, the adrenaline hits and you jerk back your foot, even before the rest of your brain thinks, "SNAKE!"

It's not just about what you see. Interpersonal space between human beings has a kind of 'texture,' which we perceive through both physical and emotional reactions. Paradoxically, many of us get 'skilled' at tuning out those signals, treating them as a kind of unwanted 'noise.'

One way, therefore, to develop your intuition is to become more aware of the signals our bodies send us. Being mindful of the space between you and others can give you an early warning system that a situation is becoming potentially explosive. If someone is aggressive, psychotic, excited, depressed, menacing, hateful, is trying to con you—any 'strong' interaction—the survival brain recognizes a pattern and responds with physical reactions. There are no rules to these physical reactions: they are individual to you.

For example:
- When in proximity to the scared person, perhaps you feel warmth in your chest.
- With the con-man, your lips compress and neck tightens.
- With psychotic people, you feel a sensation of cold in your stomach
- Your hands and jaw clench with aggressive people.

Some of your physical reactions may be unpleasant or unflattering to your own self-image. For example, let us imagine that you get somewhat sick to your stomach when facing an aggressive person, or experience a subtle, but real sense of disgust when dealing with someone who is depressed. You don't need to change this reaction—it's your individualized warning system, not a mark of character. For example, you are talking with a patient and you notice that previously mentioned sense of disgust. Although he is smiling, perhaps talking fast, you know that this physical sensation happens to you very often when dealing with depressed and despairing individuals. So you shift the conversation to assess if they are depressed, because a sense of hopelessness and helplessness, the hallmarks of that state of mind, can lead to either suicidal or homicidal thoughts.

If you continue to hone your awareness in this matter, you will develop a specialized form of intuition called **MINDFULNESS**. Mindfulness is the ability to be **consciously** aware of what is going on in your interactions with another person.

Where these reactions really come in handy is when someone is trying to hide their intentions: smiling, for example, while trying to get close enough to assault with their hands or a weapon. Let's imagine, for example, a woman whom you helped when her baby choked on food. Your 'thinking mind' tells you, "She wouldn't want to hurt me! I saved her baby's life!" But your eyes are tightening and you're getting the same tension in your lower back that you have had on every occasion when someone has attacked you in the past. Don't talk yourself out of it! Danger is about to hit you right in the gut.

Figure 7.3 Honing intuition

It is easy to train yourself to become more intuitive. Simply carry a small notebook in your pocket. If you encounter anyone who interacts with you in a significant way (aggressive, manipulative, depressed, etc.), note down (later) how your body reacts. After some time, you will recognize such physical reactions as early warning signals of the other person's state of mind.

By being aware of physical sensations, you're training yourself to recognize the patterns, consciously, that your survival brain notices, unconsciously. Instead of concluding "I was having a lucky day. Something told me not to knock on that door," you say, "I had that feeling in my hands I always get right before a fight. I knew something was going to happen, so I went around the back and looked in the window, and saw him standing behind the door with a piece of rebar."

Lesson #11 – Awareness of the Meaning of the Warning Signals from Body And Emotions Saves Lives

Figure 7.4 Don't label feelings—associate them with specific situations

We should be far more concerned with physical sensations than what we normally refer to as 'feelings,' our *description* of emotional states. For example, you have a sensation of high energy, with tension in your stomach. Some would call this 'anxiety,' while others would call this 'anticipation.' If you think that a sense of anxiety does not 'fit' the situation you are in, you will tend to ignore the physical sensation, or talk yourself out of it, saying such phrases to yourself as—"I'm being silly. There's no reason to be 'nervous' here."

If, on the other hand, you merely associate a physical sensation with a situation, i.e., "Every time someone tries to con me, I get a little smile and tension in my neck," you will notice your physical reactions without biasing them based on what you *think* you should feel.

Figure 7.5 Author's Experience: WARNING—when intuition was not heeded

An individual once thanked me profusely at the end of our meeting. Instead of the warm pride I get when I've helped someone (and I HAD helped him), I had a very strong reaction that I always have when someone overtly threatens me. I mentally brushed it aside, thinking, "I'm being an idiot. The man just complimented me." Sometime later, he poisoned me. I am only alive today because he chose to degrade me by contaminating my food rather than putting something lethal in it. I learned in the ugliest way possible to always pay attention to what my body 'tells' me. The body is linked to structures in the brain that serve to protect us from danger through pattern recognition rather than verbal cognitions. To treat our bodily reactions with disrespect is to disavow that which has kept humanity alive for millennia.

CHAPTER 8

Circular Breathing—Be The Eye In The Center Of The Hurricane

Aggression and violence can smash through a previously peaceful day with the force of a hurricane. However, when you can respond by stepping coolly into the worst of situations, you embody the eye of the hurricane, with all the chaos coalescing and revolving around you. The root of this skill lies in breath control. Using a method called 'circular breathing,' you regain control of your physical self. When you control your body, you control your life. Then you're in a position to take control of the crisis as well as the person causing it.

Figure 8.1 Tactical breathing is not 'blissing out'

Lest there be any confusion—This is NOT a "time-out" where you take a few deep breaths and then return to the patient (or burning building), refreshed. You are training your body and mind to go into this breathing as an automatic response to danger and stress, one that should be instantaneous. And remember—you can still be moving very fast while breathing very slowly.

Unlike my younger days when the adrenalin would hit and I'd start breathing fast and high in the chest, these days, my breathing usually slows down in emergency situations. You are practicing to develop a 'pseudo-instinct'—a trained response so bone-deep that you don't even have to think about it; anymore than you have to tell yourself to yank your hand from a hot stove.

Two Variations

Circular breathing is derived from East Asian martial traditions and was used to keep warriors calm on the battlefield. There are two variations. Try both, alternating between them, until you know which one works best for you. From that point on, exclusively practice the one you prefer. *If you train regularly, it will kick in automatically, rather than being something you must think about.* In essence, your breath itself becomes your center: not your body posture, not the situation in which you find yourself, or whatever is going on between you and the aggressor.

Circular Breathing Method #1 – Initial Practice Method

- Sit comfortably, feet on the floor, hands in your lap.
- Sit relaxed, but upright. Don't slump or twist your posture.
- Keep your eyes open. (**As you practice, so you will do.** If you practice with your eyes closed, your newly trained nervous system will send an impulse to close your eyes in emergency situations. If you want to use a breathing method for closed-eye guided imagery or relaxation—to get *away* from your problems, so to speak—use another method altogether.)
- Breathe in through the nose.
- Imagine the air traveling in a line down the front of your body to a point 2 inches below the navel.
- Momentarily pause, letting the breath remain in a dynamic equilibrium.
- As you exhale, imagine the air looping around your lower body, between your legs and up through the base of your spine.
- Continue to exhale, imagine the air going up your spine and around your head and then out of your nose.
- *NOTE: If nasal breathing is impaired, you can breathe through your mouth. Keep the mouth only a little open, so that the breath enters and exits in a controlled fashion*

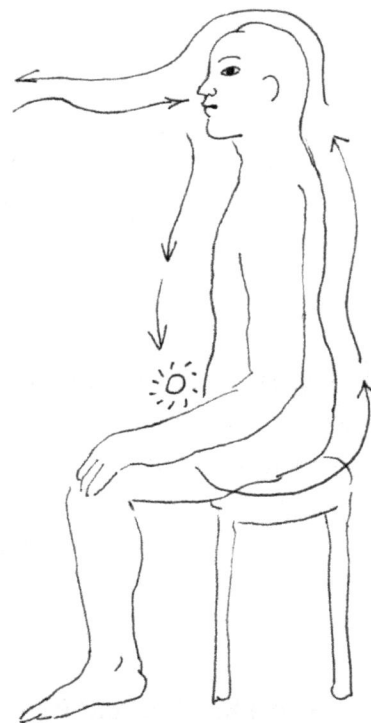

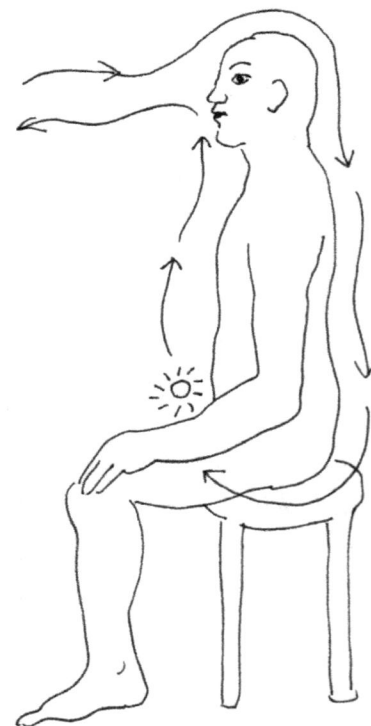

Circular Breathing Method #2 – Initial Practice Method

- Sit comfortably, feet on the floor, hands in your lap.
- Sit relaxed, but upright. Don't slump or twist your posture
- Keep your eyes open. (**As you practice, so you will do.** If you practice with your eyes closed, your newly trained nervous system will send an impulse to close your eyes in emergency situations. If you want to use a breathing method for closed-eye guided imagery or relaxation—so get *away* from your problems, so to speak—use another method altogether.)
- Breathe in through the nose.
- Imagine the air going up around your head, looping down the back, falling down each vertebra, continuing down past the base of the spine to the perineum, and continuing up the front of the body to a point 2 inches below the navel.
- Momentarily pause, letting the breath remain in a dynamic equilibrium.
- As you exhale, imagine the air ascending up the centerline of your body and out your nose.
- *NOTE: If nasal breathing is impaired, you can breathe through your mouth. Keep the mouth only a little open, so that the breath enters and exits in a controlled fashion*

How to Practice Circular Breathing

Some people find that imagining their breath has light or color to be helpful. Others take a finger or object to trace a line down and around the centerline of the body to help focus their attention. Choose whichever works better for you.

When you first practice, do so while seated and balanced. Once you develop some skill, try circular breathing standing, leaning, or even while driving. Most people find that after a short period of time they don't need to visualize the circulation of the breath. You literally will *feel* it, a ring of energy running through your body. You will increasingly feel balanced and ready for anything.

Once you're comfortable with your chosen pattern of breathing, experiment with it in slightly stressful circumstances, like being stuck in traffic while you have an important meeting, dealing with yet another call-out to a manipulative individual who claims illness to use the ambulance as a taxi service to a downtown hospital, or sitting through a meeting as a supervisor drones on about new paperwork requirements. Through practicing circular breathing in these slightly aggravating or anxiety-provoking situations, you will train your brain to associate this breathing with stress. You will naturally shift to this type of breathing in an emergency situation. It you have practiced enough, it kicks in by itself. There will no longer be a need to tell yourself to 'do' circular breathing. It will become automatic, replacing old patterns of breathing that actually increased anxiety or anger within you.

When Should You Use Circular Breathing

The way you organize physically affects your thinking. For example, if you let your body slump, breathe shallowly and start sighing, you will actually start to feel depressed. If you clench your fists and start glaring around with a lot of tension in your body, you will start to feel angry. (You have probably observed a number of patients working themselves up in just this way.) Similarly, circular breathing creates its own mindset: one adaptable and ready for anything, equally prepared for an easy conversation or a fight, yet fixed on neither.

This method of breathing is very helpful when you're anticipating a potentially dangerous situation: anything from driving towards someone's residence in a gang-infested area, to getting a call about a child who has a history of previous cardiac events. This breathing activates the entire nervous system in a way that enhances both creativity and the ability to survive.

Even in the middle of a confrontation, particularly a verbal one, there are many times when this breathing will have a very powerful effect on both yourself and others. People tend to template their mood to the most powerful individual close by. Not only do we get more stressed or upset in the presence of an upset person, but also we become more peaceful in the presence of a calm one. We are sure that you know first responders who, when they walk onto a scene, often calm it down before they have said a word. You have probably seen the opposite as well, firefighters or EMTs who fire everyone up without saying a word. Using this breathing method is a vital tool in making you the former type—an individual of quiet power.

Use this method of breathing after the crisis as well. You need to regroup to go on with the rest of your shift. Circular breathing will bring you back to a calm and relaxed state, prepared to handle the next crisis, should one occur.

The crisis may not end at the end of your shift. If we bring feelings from a crisis situation back home, we carry violence back to our family. Therefore, before entering your home, sit quietly in your car or even in the yard (or if your neighborhood isn't safe, let your family know you need to go to a quiet area before really 'coming home') and practice this breathing for a moment or two. The only thing that should come home is 'you,' not the crises you have weathered.

Lesson #12 – Circular Breathing Saves Lives

Circular Breathing to Ward Off or Even Heal from Trauma

> **Figure 8.2 Note on circular breathing to ward off trauma**
> Although the material in this section may seem a little to 'therapy' oriented to some, it is invaluable if you ever find yourself having difficulty dealing with a traumatic reaction and help is either not available, or you can't or shouldn't avail yourself of the help that is offered. Keep this in reserve for when you need it.

Post-Traumatic Stress Disorder (PTSD) is not defined by how horrible the event sounds to others. It is defined by the victim's response to the event. PTSD is not exactly a problem of memory; it is a problem because the event has not fully *become* a memory. Instead, it is still experienced as if it is happening in present time. When an event is fully a memory, it is experienced as something in the past, over and done with. Another way to think of it is a scar; it may not be pretty, and it certainly is a sign that something significant happened, but it no longer hurts. A trauma, on the other hand, is an open wound. It is an *experience*. It is not in the past: it may be affect every moment of the person's life, or suddenly emerge when evoked by something that elicits a sense that the event is happening again.

In PTSD the person's nervous system is set to react as if there is an emergency whenever the trauma is recalled. This can be anything from an explicit memory to a small reminder. For example, although unconscious of the reason, an EMT gets anxious every time someone coughs—because, for example, one of his team coughed right before they found the dead child, or the floor in the burning building gave way. Image-associated breathing techniques, which affect the brain as a whole, can assist people in realizing that the event is over, no longer part of one's current life.

Figure 8.3 Flash images versus traumatic images

It is not uncommon for firefighters and EMTs to encounter a stimulus (a sound, smell or location) that is somehow associated with an extreme situation, and see a 'flash image' of the event. This can be very startling the first time this happens. It is important in our high-stress field to distinguish what is a common bi-product of an event, one that will recede over time, and what is more severe, such as having the image occur incessantly and feeling imprisoned by it.

The following should be helpful in handing PTSD:

1. If you have been traumatized, whenever you think about the event (or it forcibly intrudes into your consciousness), your body tenses or twists in various ways. Your breathing pattern often changes. If you physically organize (with your breath, muscular tension, posture, etc.) *as if* something is happening, the brain believes that it truly is occurring right now. This is PTSD.

2. If this is your situation, go someplace where you won't be disturbed for a while. Make the mental image of that trauma as vivid as you can tolerate. This takes some courage, because most of us *simultaneously* 'avoid-as-we-remember.' If only for a moment or two, meet it head on. Notice, in *fine de*tail, how you physically and emotionally react. As difficult as this may be, it is important to establish for yourself what your baseline response is to the trauma. You must clearly experience what it 'does' to you when you recollect it. (NOTE: if this is too difficult to do by yourself, do so with a trusted friend. They are not there to offer advice, or even speak at all. They are there to lend their human support, silently, as you work this thing out).

3. Now take a couple of deep sighs. Sighing breaks up patterns of muscular tension and respiration. This is like rebooting your computer when the program is corrupt.

4. Mentally say to the ugly experience: "Move right over there to my (right or left). I'll get to you in a minute." For some people, it is even helpful to make a physical gesture, 'pushing' the experience off to the side. You won't be able to *force* yourself to stop thinking about an experience if it has psychological power. Instead, move it aside, as if you are guiding a wounded person to a waiting room, while you organize yourself to properly deal with it.

5. Now initiate your preferred method of circular breathing.

6. As the memory creeps back in (and it will), just breathe and center yourself, again placing the memory off to the side. Once again say, "I'll get to you in a minute." You can't fight it, so don't try. Just ease it aside until you are ready.

7. When your breathing is smooth and your body is centered, you will be relaxed like an athlete, ready to move, but with no wasted effort or unnecessary tension.

8. Now, deliberately bring that ugly memory or trauma into your thoughts and imagination. As you again find yourself reacting, continue circular breathing, trying to bring yourself back to physical balance as you maintain focus on the traumatic memory.

9. Bit by bit, in either one session or a few, you will notice that you are increasingly able to hold the image with a relaxed body and a balanced posture. You are now able to re-experience the memory

without the same painful, tense, or distorted response you had in the past. You are, metaphorically speaking, turning the open wound into scar tissue. You are not wiping the slate of memory clean. Rather, you are placing it in a proper context—something that happened to you, but does not define you.

Lesson #13 – Letting Go (Turning Wounds into Scars) Saves Lives

Figure 8.4 Doing for yourself

What is particularly valuable to many firefighters and EMTs is that it allows one to take power back on one's own. There is no doubt that counseling can be invaluable. However, it is sometimes hard to find a good counselor who understands a firefighter or EMT's situation. There are also times when a CISM is not appropriate for a first responder, either due to his or her own character ('I do for myself'), or the particular situation. This is particularly true if a CISM is mandated by policy. Being forced to participate in a CISM or counseling session can be counter-productive; it may even exacerbate the trauma.

If one can, on a daily basis, 'inoculate' oneself against stressful, even potentially traumatic experiences, life will continue to be enjoyable, or will become enjoyable once again, even as you continue working in a highly stressful environment. The goal is not trying to restore some kind of mythic 'innocence' that one had 'pre-trauma.' The goal is to relegate the experience to its proper place—something ugly that happened sometime in the past.

CHAPTER 9

The Intoxication And Joy
Of Righteous Anger

Most people consider anger to be a harmful emotion, one that upsets the angry person as well as the recipient. For many, if not most people, anger feels unpleasant as well. This isn't true for everyone. There is a subset of people, including some firefighters and EMTs, who don't mind anger or even fighting whatsoever, particularly when they believe their cause is just. These individuals go off-center in an interesting way, becoming calm, even happy, when someone offends them. As a boxer once stated in regards to an opponent, "When he gets hurt, he wants the round to be over. When I get hurt, I get happy." Such people, when functioning in a professional capacity, have an especially difficult task. They must recognize that when they feel *good*, they're in danger of becoming part of the problem. Instead of imposing calm, they escalate the situation, not minding it in the least.

Circular breathing (Chapter 8), for those who are anxious, stressed, or frightened provides a real sense of peace and relief. However, if confrontation feels good to you, calming breathing seems like the last thing you would like to do. If you feel righteously enraged, you feel good! You think, "Center myself? Hell, no. I'm right where I want to be."

This isn't about becoming some sort of sage: never angered, never off-balance. There are times when you *should* be angry—it may even help to keep you alive. The real issue here is the firefighter or EMT who reacts angrily to even the slightest provocation, or worse, one who treats aggravating or troublesome people with contempt and disrespect, because they are looking for the 'high' of aggression. Such righteously angry first responders escalate minor situations into serious ones—heightening the likelihood of a physical altercation with the patient, they place everyone involved in unnecessary danger.

The righteously angry first responder may be known among his or her peers for this type of reaction, but he or she is also the one most likely to *not* recognize this, and *not* believe they need to do anything to correct it. If this description fits, your task is to recognize the special joy that comes with righteous anger, and bring yourself to a calm state of mind, even though in the heat of the angry moment, it feels like a loss rather than a gain.

Protecting Your Family From What You Otherwise Would Bring Home

Another type of righteous anger is that evoked when someone does something so clearly evil that one feels annihilation of the perpetrator is the only justifiable response. Returning to the subject of the last chapter, this is a particularly important example of how such breathing can protect your family. For example, both of us (authors) have had the experience of feeling utterly contaminated by being in the presence of the perpetrators of child abuse or sexual assault. Conforming to our professional commitments, we have rendered such individuals assistance. But we have each left the individual, feeling we have failed because we did not take their throat between our hands and squeeze the life out of them.

Both of us made sure that we never brought this feeling home. Each of us had the experience of sitting in our car, running the breath around our body, maybe going to a quiet place in the house or yard and working through the images in our brains so that when we walked into the presence of our spouse and children, the only thing each of us ever brought home was ourselves. No child molester or other evildoer will ever walk into the house with us.

Lesson #14 – Protecting Our Family From The Ugliness Of The Job Protects The Quality Of All Our Lives

Figure 9 Lifesaving Points in Section II

Lesson #6 – Centering Saves Lives

Lesson #7 – Peer Support Saves Lives

Lesson #8 – Intuition Saves Lives

Lesson #9 – Being Cool Saves Lives

Lesson #10 – Awareness of Interpersonal Space Saves Lives

Lesson #11 – Awareness of the Meaning of the Warning Signals from Body And Emotions Saves Lives

Lesson #12 – Circular Breathing Saves Lives

Lesson #13 – Letting Go (Turning Wounds into Scars) Saves Lives

Lesson #14 – Protecting Our Family From The Ugliness Of The Job Protects The Quality Of All Our Lives

SECTION III

Dealing With Unusual, Intense, and Eccentric Communication Styles

CHAPTER 10

A Reminder—Deal With The Behavior, Not The Cause

What is a mental illness? Is it any odd or eccentric behavior, or should we confine the term for more serious disturbances. It sometimes seems that we lump together mental phenomena that are as disparate as the distinction between a common cold and lung cancer. Yes, both may be troublesome, and make breathing difficult, but they are profoundly different disorders. Nonetheless, it is more difficult to communicate with anyone who displays unusual or eccentric patterns of behavior, and without ability to effectively communicate with a patient, they are at greater medical risk.

It is not incumbent upon firefighters and EMTs, however, to diagnose what mental disorder a patient may be suffering, even in the most general way. This book—and firefighter and EMT responsibility—focuses on behavior, not on specific mental illness. Even so, if someone behaves in a way that makes it difficult to communicate with them, or even more problematically, exhibits disruptive behaviors, then you should be prepared with several skills:

- The ability to recognize a pattern of behavior that may present a danger to the patient or to others.
- The knowledge of best practice communication strategies to respond to a person who is displaying such a pattern of behavior, whatever the cause may be.

Figure 10 – People are not 'one thing'

It is also important to remember that each behavior—each chapter—describes a behavior, not a 'type.' Many individuals may exhibit several behaviors: for example, a person may show delusions, paranoia and concrete thinking.

CHAPTER 11

Rigid Personality

Some patients may possess normal or even superior intelligence, yet they have tremendous difficulty negotiating social interactions. Often diagnosed with Asperger's Syndrome or 'High Functioning Autism,' they find other people to be incomprehensible, confusing, or threatening. They find it very difficult to know from other's facial expressions, body posture, and vocal tone, what they're feeling or thinking. Others, particularly some with schizophrenia, show a similar combination of 'social cluelessness' and rigidity in communication with others. Such rigid patients become fixated on their own preoccupations, and imagine that everyone else shares them. They can also be very literal (concrete) and they can get stuck on certain thoughts and behaviors (obsessive). Others are simply not interested in or aware of others' feelings. This can lead them to be very blunt, or brutally honest.

Figure 11.1 Examples of socially clueless statements by a patient displaying rigid personality traits

1. "What is the bump on your face? It's quite ugly. You know, it could be a melanoma, which could cause your face to simply rot away, or it could infect your brain and then you'd die. I've seen photos of tumors that have actually eaten right through a person's cheek and you can see their teeth and tongue out the side of their face."

2. "You've gained a lot of weight in the last year. I don't mind, but many men don't think that is attractive."

They have no malevolent intent. Other people's feelings—unimaginable and incomprehensible—are simply not relevant data to the person.

Such people often don't appear to be mentally ill. Rather, they're stiff and socially awkward, always a little out-of-sync. Their voice may be too loud, and they may sound odd. Their eye contact may be 'off,' or non-existent, and they are sometimes physically uncoordinated. They don't pay attention to the effect that their actions or appearance might have on others, and they are frequently insensitive to body spacing.

Because they find people unpredictable and unreadable, they are frequently very anxious. Some, therefore, use self-soothing movements, like flapping their hands or rhythmically tapping an object or body part to help distract them from what is stressful. One thing that can make individuals with rigid personality particularly dangerous to fire fighters and EMTs is that many such people react violently to physical touch.

Rather than trying to establish an empathic connection, 'quoting the rules' with such a patient is often the best option. Attempts to validate such patient's feelings, on the other hand, will merely result in them becoming increasingly confused or upset. Consider this: if the firefighter or EMT's body language, tone of voice, and facial expression are incomprehensible, the rules, clearly stated, will be very reassuring. State each rule in a matter-of-fact way, as if simply providing information. Follow this up with a logical sequence of steps to solve their problem. You must be as concrete and literal as they are. State the obvious. For example:

- She says, "Why should I lower my voice? I'm angry!"
- Your reply should be, "Because it is a rule when speaking with an EMT that you inform them of your condition with a quiet voice."
- "That's a stupid rule," she replies.
- "Nonetheless," you return, "it is the rule." They may, then, ask you for exceptions. "Am I allowed to raise my voice if you administer some violent treatment without anesthesia?" They feel the need to cover all possibilities. However, after too many questions, you must take over and give a general policy that, hopefully, will cover all variations

Figure 11.2 De-escalation of someone with rigid personality traits

Pavel. "I can't go to the hospital now. I saw seven orb spiders in my house, and that is bad destiny."

Firefighter/EMT. "Pavel, with your medical condition, you must go to the hospital, no matter what number of spiders you have seen."

Pavel. "But this could mean a disaster for someone. Seven spiders is terrible."

Firefighter/EMT. "The rule is that people with the symptoms you are showing must go to the hospital when told by a firefighter or EMT to do so, and this applies even when you believe that there are unlucky signs."

Pavel. "Destiny, not bad luck."

Firefighter/EMT. "It is still the rule, be it destiny or not. The rule has no deviation."

Pavel. "How about if a meteor hits the hospital?"

Firefighter/EMT. "Pavel, the rule is ironclad. If you are told to go, you must.

Pavel. "Well, I think that's very irresponsible, that you would take someone to the hospital when a meteor might hit!"

Firefighter/EMT. "Pavel, get your coat now. It's time to go. That IS the rule, based on medical knowledge."

Figure 11.3 Review: dealing with rigid personality

You will recognize the person with a rigid personality because they get stuck on things that seem rather odd in the circumstances. They seem unaware of their effect on others. Their emotions—if they're even displaying any—aren't those you would expect given the emergency or physical discomfort they are obviously suffering.

- State the rules in a matter-of-fact way, as if simply providing information.
- Follow this up with a logical sequence of steps to solve their problem.
- Discussion about their feelings will be counter-productive. Tactical paraphrasing (Chapter 45) ordinarily used to deal with an angry person tend to make things worse.
- Be aware that they may react with fear, anxiety or rage to body contact.
- Don't get deflected from your task. Like a parody of a lawyer, they may bring up possible exceptions to your order. Remember, though, that they are not playing games. 'Step through' the objections, and simply state that they're required to follow the rule.
- Use this type of strategy only when it is clear that you are interacting with a rigid individual: stiff, concrete, and socially out of sync. Think of Data on Star Trek: either coldly logical, or if they become confused—frustrated and out of control.

CHAPTER 12

Tell It Like It Is—Communication With Concrete Thinkers

Concrete thinkers have a lot of difficulty understanding metaphors, slang, or imagery. Instead, they take everything you say literally. For example:

- "Way to go!" an expression meant as praise. The concrete patient thinks, "Where?"
- "Get out of my face," an expression that means that the person shouldn't be oppositional or aggressive. The concrete patient thinks, "How can someone be inside someone's flesh?"

When communicating with concrete thinkers, Firefighters and EMTs should use short, clear sentences, with simple, specific words that are easy to understand. Remember, they can comply with a specific command, but not even understand the general principal. Beyond the specific of what you say, your tone is important as well—speak in a firm manner, but do not show much emotion. If you become angry or frustrated, the concrete patient will react to your emotions, not your instructions.

Figure 12.1 Example of ineffective and effective dialogue between a firefighter/EMT and a concrete thinker

Firefighter/EMT. "Okay. So you don't have to worry anymore."

Concrete Person. "I wasn't worried. I was upset."

Firefighter/EMT. "Oh, okay, you were upset. Anyway, the ambulance is coming, and will be here shortly. I want you to sit tight."

Concrete Person. "How do I sit tight? Should I wrap myself in a blanket?"

Firefighter/EMT. *(Sigh)* "No, you don't have to wrap yourself up. I meant you should sit quietly and...."

Concrete Person. "You mean I shouldn't talk?"

Firefighter/EMT. *(Aghhhhh)* "No, you can talk! It's a figure of speech!"

We think you get the idea. Let us take this last example and show what might be a better way to accomplish the task. Imagine this just from the Firefighter or EMT 's side:

- "The ambulance is coming."
- "Sit in the chair right here."
- "Yes, sit where you are right now and keep talking to me."
- "Yes, I can hear them too. No, don't wait by the door. Sit in the chair until they come in the house."

Figure 12.2 Review: concrete thinkers

You will recognize *concrete thinkers* because they take what you say literally. Therefore be sure to:

- Use clear, short sentences, with a firm, calm voice.
- Give directions using simple words that are easy to understand.
- Show a minimum of emotion. Don't get irritated when they don't immediately understand you. They respond much more to your tone of voice than to what you say.

CHAPTER 13

Information Processing And Retention— Consolidating Gains

Many mentally ill people develop the ability to 'fake normal.' People around them may do frightening things, but they don't show their fear. Other people may anger them, but they smile and pretend everything is all right. Conversations and ideas may be too complex, too fast, or irrelevant to what is going on inside them, but they have learned to pick up the rhythm of other people's speech, nod at the right moments, smile or laugh when needed, and agree with the tag lines that invite such agreement.[12]

Never assume, therefore, that a mentally ill person understands what you have told them just because they nod their head at the right moment. You need to verify what they've understood:

- **The least effective method is for you to repeat yourself using other words.** If they have either tuned you out, or didn't understand you the first time, they may fake understanding again. This is different from the repetition you must do with the disorganized patient, when you DO repeat yourself when giving instructions (Chapter 22). Here, you're checking to see if what you said got through. However, simply repeating your instructions, and assuming the other person understood what you said is often a mistake.

- **Have them repeat your instructions.** However, some patients echo what you say, so this doesn't prove that they actually understand or will follow through.

- **Another method is open sentences.** For example, "So, Diane, if I've got it right, you will take your medicine in one hour. And tomorrow you will…." (If she understands, she will fill in the rest of the sentence.)

- **Write down the most important points.** Many mentally ill people don't assimilate a lot of information that they hear, no matter how hard they listen. It is sometimes useful to pull out a small card and write down the most important points of the conversation or agreement. Give them the card, go over the items, and tell them to check the card if they have any difficulty remembering what they're supposed to do. (We're aware that there are many circumstances where this strategy would be out of the question, but both of us have used it on occasion.)

Figure 13 Review of consolidation of gains

- The least effective way is to repeat yourself, hoping that their replies and head-nods really mean that they understood you.
- Have the person repeat back your instructions.
- Use open sentences and questions, allowing the person to fill in the blanks.
- Write down the most important points on a card.

CHAPTER 14

Coping With Stubborn Refusals

There are many occasions where you are treating your patient with respect—at least you've started out that way. The patient, however, sets her heels. She won't take her medications, fill out paperwork, go to the doctor, or any one of a number of issues.

Of course, if you have been bossing her around, patronizing her, or treating her with disrespect, it isn't surprising if she resists you. All people, mentally ill or not, have pride, and no one likes another person talking down to them or controlling their lives. However, once you're clear that it isn't your approach that is creating the problem, what, if anything, can you do?

Figure 14 Steps to compliance

- **Focus on the task.** It is very important NOT to take the impasse personally. If you do, it just adds additional problems to work out between you.
- **Clarify the message using a calm commanding voice.** Be clear on what you require the person to do now. Stay very concrete.
- **Control the interview.** Stay on topic and don't allow the person to divert your attention to unrelated issues.
- **Dispassionately state the consequences**. This pertains to the medical consequences of refusal, or what the Firefighter or EMT will do (leave, for example) in response.
- **Place the power in their hands.** Again, in situations where this is a question of the person complying with a medical necessity, step back emotionally and sometimes physically (a fraction of a step). Say something like, "You are absolutely correct. You can refuse, and we'll leave. Your infection will get worse. Or you can accept treatment and probably be walking without pain in a few days. Looks like you have a decision to make."

CHAPTER 15

Coping With Repetitive Demands, Questions, And Obsessions

Sometimes mentally ill patients make a repetitive demand for information that you have already answered or explained in exhaustive detail. There can be a variety of reasons for this, and each should be dealt with in a different manner:

- They get 'stuck' on an obsessive idea. No matter how many times they get an answer to their concern, they 'have to' ask it again. This is often a sign of Obsessive-Compulsive Disorder (OCD). Such people experience unbearable anxiety when they don't give in to the obsession (fixated thought) or compulsion (an unshakable drive/demand to do something). Be aware that they may feel so trapped by their compulsions that they lash out if they believe themselves to be impeded in carrying them out. Given that you are attending to a medical emergency, you must calmly require them to do what is necessary to comply with your directives, while keeping fully aware of the potential for assault. In situations where the compulsion is not dangerous, you can tell them that they can fulfill the compulsion *after* they comply with you, as in, "You can count the holes in the ceiling after you give me your arm, so I can take your blood pressure." In other cases, you can allow them to fulfill the compulsion in order to engender more compliance, such as, "You can wash your hands, one time, and then I will check your pulse. I will use sterile gloves, but you are welcome to wash your hands again afterwards." However, be aware that some compulsive people never do a 'good enough' job, and they will feel compelled to do it again and again. In this case, go back to the first choice, and insist on compliance first.

- Others obsess as part of a disorder like schizophrenia, developmental disability, intoxication, or other serious impairments of cognition. If they are (re) asking the question because they either forgot or didn't understand the answer, it is most reasonable to answer them again. If they are not able to retain the information, their repetitive questions or obsessing on a single point may be due to information processing errors (Chapter 13). These patients are not playing games; they simply have cognitive deficits that cripple their ability to understand and/or retain information.

- Sometimes people repeat a question *intending* to be irritating or challenging. Say in a matter-of-fact tone, "You already know the answer to that," or otherwise point out that they already have the information and *move on*. By disengaging, you are implicitly saying, "I'm not participating in the game." You are thereby informing them that continued game playing will impede them from getting the services they are requesting (or demanding).

Figure 15.2 Dealing with repetitive demands and compulsions

- If the person is obsessive-compulsive in behavior, either offer them a chance to fulfill the (non-dangerous) compulsion after they comply with your requirements, or in some cases, allow them to fulfill the compulsion first and then they will comply. If they get stuck, and can neither fulfill the compulsion or let it go for a time, take over calmly and require them to comply with you first. However, do be prepared in case they become assaultive if they become frustrated in response to your directive.

- With psychotic or other seriously mentally ill people who get stuck on something, remember that it is not game playing. It is due to their cognitive impairments. It is usually easier to simply answer the question again and move on.

- For those who are playing games, simply reply, "You already know the answer to that," and move on with your task.

CHAPTER 16

The Need For Reassurance

Some people are quite anxious by nature or circumstances. For others, intolerable anxiety is either their primary illness, a side effect of either their medication or some illicit drug they are taking, or one of the most troublesome symptoms of their mental disorder. **Anxiety is living as if something that you're afraid might happen in the future is happening right now.** For example, the person reads about an earthquake in Japan, imagines what might happen to his/her town if an earthquake hit, and suddenly they are afraid as if the ground has started shaking.

When dealing with someone afflicted by anxiety, you must draw a graceful line. Don't coddle the person: if you treat him/her like they are weak, they will believe you and become even more anxious, relying on you to assuage their feelings. They may think that something awful is going to happen, and that is why you're talking in such careful tones. At the same time, don't affect a cheerful, "ain't no big thing" tone of voice. This kind of falsity will make the person either uneasy or irritated. Instead, make your voice matter-of-fact. Take their anxiety into account, but speak with an expectation that they're strong enough to manage what they must do.

Figure 16 The anxious person

The reassurance that you can offer anxious people need is not about the facts about their future concerns. Rather, reassurance is embodied in your demeanor—a confident voice that makes the person feel stronger for listening.

CHAPTER 17

Dealing With People
With Extreme Mood Swings

People with mood swings display behavior that is sometimes referred to as labile. They're angry one minute, sad the next, and happy a couple minutes later. You commonly see such behaviors among those patients with borderline personality disorder, bipolar disorder, or those who have incurred neurological damage through head-injury, infection, birth defects or long-term substance abuse. They can be very difficult to communicate with, much less de-escalate, because just as you try to deal with their current emotions, they shift into another. They can be verbally abusive, provocative, complaining, passive-aggressive, blaming, apologetic, ingratiating, and friendly all in the space of an hour. They often attempt to get control of you even when they have no control over themselves.

Coping with Mood Swings

Rather than reacting to the person's behavior with body language or words that manifest your own anger or frustration, remain balanced and emotionally non-reactive. **You influence them by being exactly what they are not.** The more you're unaffected by their emotional storms, the more likely that they will calm down (Section II)

Figure 17 Review: mood swings

Patients with mood swings shift emotions rapidly, with no particular relationship to the situation they're in.

- Don't mirror the patient's emotional state, reacting to what they do.
- Control them through controlling your own emotions. Remain powerfully calm.
- Speak in a firm, yet calm, and controlled manner.
- Because they display any emotion you can imagine, use general de-escalation tactics, as described throughout the book, as needed.

CHAPTER 18

They Aren't Moving—
What To Do?

You've surely been in situations where you tell a mentally ill patient to do something, and they stare vacantly at you, voice a million questions, express misgivings or anxiety, or drift off into a monologue about something completely different. They simply won't do what **you** think is good for them. They may not even understand what that is.

Why are you frustrated? Is it out of concern for their well-being or is it because they are not complying with YOU. Before taking it personally, you have to determine if they're truly capable of doing what you think they should. Expectations must be realistic, especially with mentally ill patients.

Observe yourself as you try to get the other person 'moving.' Do you like the sound of your voice? Don't sound like a 'cheerleader' in an attempt to try to get them to comply. ("C'mon. You can do this!"). Don't betray your frustration either. Keep your dignity! Persons with mental illness are far more likely to be compliant with firefighters and EMTs whom they respect—and from whom they've received respect.

Figure 18 What to do when they aren't 'moving'
- Be aware of their limitations. Don't expect the person to do something they can't.
- If you perceive the patient is playing games, don't waste too much time asking repeatedly for them to do something. Furthermore, don't do things for them if they can do it themselves.

CHAPTER 19

Useful Tactics For Dealing With Symptoms
Of Paranoia And Persecution

Figure 19.1 This chapter focuses on paranoia, not psychosis

This chapter focuses on tactics specific to paranoia. Rather than the delusional state, which we will discuss in Chapters 24 & 25, here we are discussing an attitude with the following characteristics: a sense of being persecuted, consistent blame of others rather than oneself, and a hair-trigger sensitivity to being vulnerable.

The *delusional* paranoid patient has this attitude complicated by fixed false beliefs and even hallucinations.

Dealing with a paranoid patient can be surpassingly difficult. The person's motto of life could be summed up in a phrase: "If there is a problem here, it's your fault." The paranoid world is one of dominance and submission: the paranoid tries to dominate the other people in their lives, and is terrified or enraged at being forced to submit.

The paranoid patient (even without delusions) bears a consistent attitude of blame, resentment of authority, fear of vulnerability, and an expectation of being betrayed by people they trust. Stimulant users, notably those addicted to methamphetamine and cocaine, frequently display these behaviors. It is also a very common 'solution' that criminals arrive at to excuse any failure. Paranoid people are, at core level, terrified that they will be made vulnerable, but they're aggressive toward that of which they're afraid. One helpful image of the paranoid person is an angry porcupine: all quills, with a soft underbelly, hunched over, ready to strike in hair-trigger reaction.

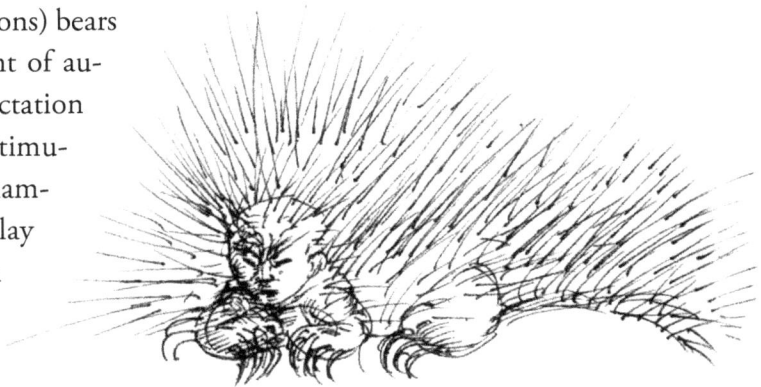

- **Paranoid people interpret relaxation as vulnerability.** Friendship means letting your guard down. Therefore, such people can become more paranoid when you begin to establish rapport with them. With paranoid folks with whom you have frequent contact, such as some homeless mentally ill patients, don't be surprised if they suddenly flare up with suspicion or accusations after an occasion that was friendly or otherwise uneventful.

- **Being mistaken is another form of vulnerability.** Rather than admitting wrongdoing or mistakes, paranoid patients reflexively *project* negative feelings on the other person. If they feel hate, they believe you hate them. If they have any difficulty with a medical intervention, they will claim you deliberately hurt them or subjected them to noxious or dangerous treatment.
- **Paranoid people live like detectives.** They continually search for evidence to prove what they already know is true. They have *ideas of reference*, in which they believe that other people's conversations, glances, or actions are directed at them. They assume that others are conspiring about them, talking about them, or laughing at them. Ironically, their (re)actions, in response to these ideas often cause others to act in exactly the way the paranoid person expects and fears.
- **Paranoid people make others uncomfortable and/or afraid.** Because of their aggressive or standoffish behavior, they can make other people uncomfortable or afraid. If they sense fear in you, however, they will expect you to attack them, and they will then 'attack you back first.' Fear drives their aggression.

Try to Let Them Know What Is Going On

- Because paranoid people are so suspicious, they will often quiz you concerning why you're doing something. It often makes tactical sense to say what you're going to do, so there is no ambiguity.
- At the same time, you shouldn't accept being quizzed incessantly. You aren't required to explain every action. In fact, it might be a tactic to throw you off guard or distract you.

Physical and Psychological Personal Space with the Paranoid Patient

Many paranoid people are preoccupied, even obsessed with fears that they will be invaded or controlled in some fashion. Those in paranoid psychotic states are often afraid that they will be molested or otherwise sexually violated. Some of the following are, of course, relevant when dealing with any patient, but they're doubly important with the paranoid patient.

- **Maintain the angle.** Whether standing or sitting, turn your body at a slight angle, so that physical 'confrontation' is a choice rather than a requirement. If you 'square off' and directly face a paranoid patient, you *force* him or her to turn away if he/she doesn't want to face you.
- **Mindfulness.** Never let down your own guard. You're in an avalanche zone, and anything could set off another slide.
- **Too friendly is as dangerous as a threat.** Try to be aware when things are getting too relaxed. It isn't only about you maintaining awareness. If the paranoid person relaxes, they may suddenly startle, realizing that for a brief moment, they let their guard down. They may respond by exploding to make sure you don't 'take them over.'
- **Cover your triggers.** Paranoid people may try to provoke you. If you lose your temper, they will feel justified in whatever they do to you as well as it keys into their terror-based aggression. A slang expression for this is 'fear biters.' They bark and snarl and when you react, they attack as if you went after them first.

Is There a Specific Paranoid Rage or Violence?

There is no specific 'paranoid rage.' Instead, paranoia is an 'engine' that drives rage in all its various forms. Verbally control the patient using tactics specific to the mode of rage they're exhibiting rather than de-escalating 'paranoia' itself. Paranoid patients can exhibit traits of fear, frustration, intimidation, and manipulation. With their focus, however, they're rarely disorganized (Section IX).

Figure 19.2 Review: paranoia and persecution

The paranoid patient has an attitude that if anything is wrong it is another person's fault. Whether delusional or not, they see others as conspiring against them or persecuting them.

- If they are also delusional and paranoid, use any of the standard tactics for delusional people. (Chapters 24 & 25)
- De-escalate based on the behavior, not the paranoia.
- Let them know what's going on.
- Speak in formal tones. Don't be too friendly.
- They will try to provoke you so they can 'hit you back first.'
- Be aware of both physical and emotional spacing. Maintain a correct distancing, neither too close nor too far.
- Differentiate by not being too friendly, and if they're delusional, clearly separate yourself from their paranoid ideas without getting into an argument with them.
- Maintain your calm—the paranoid patient is usually assaultive when they feel under attack, when they perceive you as controlling them, or when they perceive that you are afraid.
- If you do have to take them to the hospital or intervene medically on scene, let them know what is going on and why. Paranoid patient are most likely to become dangerous when they base their actions on their imagination rather than on reality.

CHAPTER 20

Dropping Stones In A Well—
Latency

Latency is a behavior that is often a manifestation of disorganization (Chapter 22), but because of both its significance and its confusing nature, we have chosen to discuss it as an entity of its own. This is a behavior in which people respond to communication in a much delayed manner. You ask a question, and they talk to themselves quietly as they puzzle out what you might be saying. Perhaps instead, they don't even make eye-contact, and engage in odd movements. Some latent folks may simply stare away, a vacuous look on their faces.

Figure 20.1 How to recognize latency

You will recognize latency when the person to whom you are speaking not only delays his/her answers for a long time, but also when they do reply, their communication is somewhat odd and disjointed, not really responding to the questions asked. This is different from being silent or defying you. You will get the sense that they're not 'there'—it is clearly about something going on inside of them, and not you at all.

Imagine your words to be like a stones dropping into a well. If things go as expected, you hear a splash as each stone hits the water. Now, imagine the latent mind like an old well with bricks sticking out, and a tangle of tree roots halfway down. Each stone hits the roots and bounces off a brick, one after the other. This time, you don't hear a splash—you hear nothing. Naturally, you start throwing more stones, one after another. You now have any number of stones bouncing around, colliding into each other, adding to your frustration and their confusion, without the first stone ever reaching the bottom of the well. All happens with the latent person is that they get more confused and overwhelmed. <u>Adding more words doesn't enhance communication with latent people.</u>

Figure 20.2 Example of a typical dialogue between a firefighter or EMT and a patient displaying latency

First Responder – "Ms. Smith, what is your Doctors name?"

Ms. Smith – responds after a prolonged period of time: "Do I have a doctor?"

First Responder – "It appears that you do based on the doctors name on your prescription bottles."

Ms. Smith – After a two to three minute delay, Ms. Smith says, "Yes, I do have a doctor."

Coping With Latency: Keep Things Simple

Although communicating with a latent patient can be frustrating, and often time consuming, the firefighter or EMT should remain calm. Indeed, any frustration or anger you display will only further confuse them. Keep your sentences and instructions short yet direct, and minimize the use of qualifiers, such as "you might" "maybe" "kind of," etc., that you ordinarily put in your sentences. Firefighters and EMTs should also try to minimize the use of hand gestures or changing facial expressions. This doesn't mean you should speak robotically, but simplicity is best.

It is useless to try to 'get through to them' by yelling or clapping your hands in front of their face. All this does is drive them further into the latent state, as they get more frightened, overwhelmed or confused by the irate professional yelling incomprehensible things at them.

Latent people usually don't need things explained in further detail; they just don't 'get it' the first time. Say the same thing again and again. This is like somehow throwing the **same** stone into the well again, reinforcing the original. Rather than adding a new stone, you have added weight to the one already dropping. Once it is 'heavy' enough, that stone can get through the roots and bricks and hit bottom.

If you aren't successful, you have actually established, better than any other method that the patient is incapable of responding to verbal communication, thus warranting an assessment by a mental health professional. In other words, 'failure' establishes how ill the person is.

Figure How 20.3 How to speak to a patient manifesting latency

- Keep your sentences short.
- Don't change your vocal tone.
- Repeat the instructions using the same words and the same tone of voice.
- Pause between sentences. Give the person time to process what you have said.
- Try to get the person to repeat back your instructions (No guarantees on this item!).

SECTION IV

Communication With Those
With Severe Mental Illness
Or Other Conditions That
Cause Severe Disability

CHAPTER 21

Overview Of Section IV

This section offers detailed descriptions of the most significant behaviors that seriously mentally ill patients may display, regardless of diagnosis. Along with each description will be suggestions for the best way to communicate with such patients. Please note a lot of the strategies in various sections overlap. Some are generally applicable, while others are specific to only one type of behavior/symptom. Just because an individual may display paranoia, for example, doesn't mean that such a patient is not also disorganized, delusional, or manic. What you're trying to develop is a range of communication tactics that cover as many situations as possible.

As the establishment of safety and the de-escalation of aggression are the primary purposes of this book, we focus on general patterns of communication and behavior, **regardless of the cause**. Mental illness, in this vein, doesn't only refer to such disorders as schizophrenia, bipolar disorder or depression. For example, intoxication can be considered a time-limited, substance-induced mental illness or character disorder, depending on its level of severity. Furthermore, beyond any medical condition, otherwise normal people can display acute, 'out of character' behaviors, evoked by severe stressors in their lives. Thus, for the sake of this discussion, substance abuse, distinct neurological disorders, as well as atypical episodes brought on by stress or other factors all can appear, functionally, as a mental illness. The cause may be relevant once medical treatment is initiated; the firefighter or EMT, however, should most emphatically focus on the behaviors, whatever the cause.

Speak to the Person, not the Illness

You're walking outside on an icy winter day. You slip suddenly and spin toward the pavement. You thrust out an arm that breaks your fall. It also breaks your right wrist. Your life, for a few weeks or months, is different. Even the simplest tasks are difficult and may require assistance. Still, even though you're inconvenienced and the injury probably changes your mood quite a bit, you're still 'you,' the same person as before your injury. In due time, your injuries will heal and the accident mostly forgotten as you continue through life. Such is not the case with mental illness.

Severe mental illness can cause mental and emotional disturbances far more profound than the temporary inconveniences brought on by physical injury. One's ability to think is distorted, and with delusions, reality is skewed. Perceptions may be bizarre, even hallucinatory. Emotions swing from high to low, or shift into realms at odds with one's immediate circumstances. Mental illness is an assault on one's entire world, but there is a still a person behind the symptoms. They are not bundles of raw emotions or distorted cognitions. Within every individual, there exists an undamaged self, untouched by their mental illness. We can choose to speak to the illness, or speak to the *person* who is ill.

Why Do They Stop Taking Their Meds?

The question has to be asked, doesn't it? Countless numbers of people are leading productive, vibrant lives thanks to psychiatric medications. Why do so many mentally ill people enter a hospital or clinic in a terrible state, and thanks to good care and medications, leave in an exponentially better condition. Soon after they leave, however, they stop taking their medications.

- **Bureaucratic obstacles.** The lack of affordable, accessible community health care is a major impediment to treatment for many patients, whose lack of insurance and medical coverage prevents them from filling their prescriptions, as well as the byzantine nature of the federal and state regulations regarding Medicaid and Social Security/Disability funding. For one example, if the mentally ill person is on Medicaid, they will be dropped if they are incarcerated for even the most minor of offenses. To get back on Medicaid (and regain access to their medications), they have to reapply, something that, without direct assistance, they may not be able to do.

- **Unwelcome side effects.** Among possible side-effects are muscle spasms, intolerable itching/crawling sensations in the limbs, tongue thrusting, tremors, impairment of sexual functioning, dry mouth, weight gain, weight loss, skin rashes and lesions, even life-threatening disorders that must be monitored through such invasive procedures as regular blood-draws, to name but a few.

- **No effect (or so it seems).** Many psychiatric medications aren't 'felt' beyond their side-effects. They don't make the person 'high,' or even 'better.' Apart from the side-effects, the person simply feels like 'himself/herself.' Feeling good, therefore, one draws the natural conclusion that the drug has done its job, or in other cases, doesn't work, and therefore can be discontinued.

- **No effect (in truth).** Many of the medications simply don't work for a person. They may have very high hopes that the medications will help, even cure them. All that they get, instead, are the side-effects.

- **The illness is better than the cure.** Sometimes, even apart from noxious side-effects, the illness can feel better than the 'cure.' Many psychotic patients find that the medications muffle or suppress delusions and/or hallucinations, but they don't make them disappear. Furthermore, the medications don't touch the belief system around the delusions. Life on medications, for such people, is like living under a sodden blanket. Their psychotic reality may be muffled, tranquilized, and constricted, but not otherwise changed. The medications may help them live a more stable, uneventful life, but just as we shake off constricting bedding when we're too hot or constricted, psychotic patients may discontinue medications, simply to have, from their perspective, air to breathe.

- **The use of illicit drugs or alcohol.** The person's use of illicit drugs and/or alcohol leads them to discontinue their prescribed medications.

- **Incapable of taking meds.** The patient is simply incapable of managing their medication regimen by themselves.

CHAPTER 22

Struggling In A Fog—
Dealing With Symptoms
Of Disorganization

Figure 22.1 Concerning enraged disorganized patients

Disorganization is a very complex subject. Many disorganized people are simply confused or disorderly, whereas others are in a state of rage. At its most extreme, this rage can manifest as excited delirium. Therefore, we must address this subject in several different chapters. See Chapter 49 for a detailed discussion of de-escalation of disorganized patients in a state of chaotic rage, including information dealing with agitated developmentally disabled people, and also Appendix C for a detailed protocol on Excited Delirium, the most severe manifestation of this condition.

Disorganization is a general term for the inability to adequately organize one's cognitions, perceptions, behaviors, and/or emotions. Intellectually disabled (developmentally disabled) patients, profoundly psychotic people, those suffering from any kind of dementia or delirium, as well as those who are severely intoxicated, all show disorganized behaviors.

Due to their cognitive limitations, developmentally disabled patients aren't skilled in problem-solving situations. Furthermore, they often lack the maturity to manage complex or frustrating circumstances (such as the emergency that brings you to the scene).

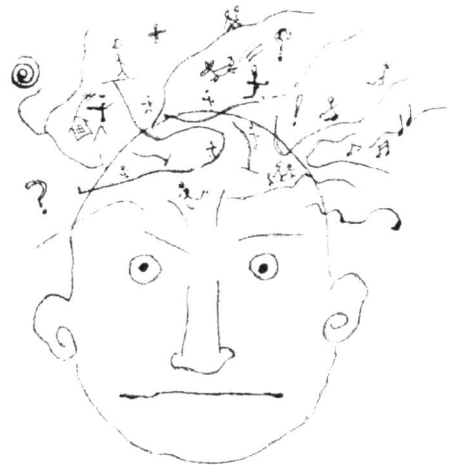

Psychotic people also become disorganized when their condition deteriorates. Oddly enough, their delusions may serve as an organizing principle, warding off chaos. For example, if you believe yourself to be surrounded by enemies or are out to save the world, you must concentrate; you are on a mission, as delusional as it may be. When one becomes disorganized, however, even one's delusions break down into chaos, often manifested in incoherent speech.

Finally, severe intoxication of any kind is a chemically induced disorganization.

> ### Figure 22.2 A Word about disorganization
>
> You will know you're dealing with a disorganized person because they are nearly incoherent, or it is otherwise impossible to communicate with them. They may seem to shift from one emotion to another for no logical reason, and it is very difficult, if not impossible, to hold their attention. Disorganization is an 'over-arching' category. A disorganized person can be latent, concrete, have mood swings, paranoia, anxiety, extreme agitation, confusion, delusions, hallucinations, and information-processing problems to name only a few. We have included specific strategies for such specific syndromes elsewhere—this chapter is concerned with the overall phenomenon.

Overstimulation

Loud noises, the presence of many people (particularly if more than one is talking), too much background noise, or bright lights (particularly the flashing lights of emergency vehicles), not only will be distracting, but may also further agitate the disorganized person. Whenever safety or time issues don't demand them, turn off your emergency lights when at the scene. While transporting the patient, do not use your siren and lights, unless they are truly necessary (when 'every second counts'). Consistent with both control and safety concerns, move the patient to a less stimulating environment whenever it is possible. **It is particularly important with disorganized people that only one person speaks to them**.

Keep It Simple

The disorganized person pays most attention to your non-verbal communication. Therefore, keep the emotion out of your voice: self-control is particularly important when de-escalating disorganized patients. Your sentences should be short, and should only have one 'packet' of information in each.

Let Me Repeat Myself

When we aren't understood, our usual impulse is to elaborate. We use different words, expressive hand and facial gestures, and we alter the emotional tone of our communication. **With disorganized people, repeat the same statement or question word-for-word.** When their disorganization is profound, you may need to do this four, five, or more times. The aim isn't to browbeat them. You shouldn't increase your volume, shouting at them to 'get through' to them. Your repetition is a touchstone of stability. Speak a little slower than normal with a 'heavy' tone, as if 'weighing down' the information so that it gets through to them.

> **Figure 22.3 General principles for communication with disorganized patients**
>
> Do not change your vocal tone or get irritated, or you will defeat the purpose of repetition. The disorganized person will react to your frustrated or angry non-verbal communication, and will become more agitated. You will undermine everyone's safety by rolling your eyes, making side-long glances of amusement, sighing, raising your voice, pointing, standing close to them to get their attention, snapping your fingers, or suddenly clapping, to name only a few maladroit strategies, whether you are repeating the same words or not.
>
> By repeating yourself several times, with a clear measured tone of voice, you have the same effect on the disorganized person as you would were you to shine a light on a footpath in the fog. By repeating yourself and telling the person exactly what you want them to do, you provide a verbal 'light' that they can focus on rather than the chaos that is otherwise overwhelming them.

Magical Thinking

Magical thinking is a term that overlaps with delusions; it is telling stories that you then believe. It is common among small children, senile and demented adults, and developmentally disabled patients. People displaying magical thinking don't show the same fixed quality of delusional people (Chapter 24), where a fundamental truth is suddenly revealed and then locked into place in the person's mind. Rather, the disorganized person verbalizes his/her fantasies, repeats them, and then believes them. It is like fable-making, the kinds of stories very young people tell, be they young in age or young in mind.

Once you've established that a claim or statement isn't true, it is non-productive to argue about magical thinking. Sometimes, just let it go. Other times, you can say, even with a little tiredness in your voice, "I've heard that story before. You don't have to tell me again." Or, "Let's not talk about that anymore."

Figure 22.4 Dealing With a Disorganized Patient

You will know you are dealing with a disorganized person when they're:

- Nearly incoherent, or otherwise impossible to communicate with;
- Shifting from one emotion to another with no logical reason;
- It is very hard, if not impossible to hold their attention;
- Acting in a bizarre or chaotic manner.

You should:

- Divide tasks into small bits;
- Give simple, specific instructions;
- Be realistic about what the person can and can't do;
- Repeat your instructions rather than elaborate on them. Don't change your vocal tone;
- Don't argue with magical thinking—redirect them to discussing what, if anything, is emergent;
- Only one person should be speaking to the disorganized person at a time.
- Whenever possible, minimize environmental distractions: the TV in the background, other people talking, even bright lights, to name just a few.

CHAPTER 23

Withdrawal From Intoxicating Substances

Figure 23.1 IMPORTANT NOTE: The question of dual diagnosis

Given our attention to various 'types' of mentally ill patients, the reader may question why we haven't devoted a large section specifically to the behaviors of 'dual-diagnosis' patients (those with both substance abuse and mental health issues) as a separate concern. There is no doubt whatsoever, that dual diagnosis can profoundly affect every aspect of a person's life. Substance abuse makes it much harder to heal from or even manage mental illness, and mental illness makes it much harder to recover from substance abuse. Furthermore, substance abuse exponentially increases the risk of violence from individuals with mental illness.

However, imagine all the descriptions of behavior necessary to distinguish between, for example, a solvent inhaling person with bipolar disorder, a marijuana smoking person with social phobia, and a schizophrenic who injects a mixture of cocaine and heroin. To be sure, each and all of these concerns are relevant when it comes to medical treatment. The only thing that we're focusing on however, is behavior that can compromise safety or emergency care. Whatever substances they may have ingested, whatever illness or syndrome they may be suffering from, we're concerned with the behaviors that they're displaying. In a crisis, **deal with the behavior, not the cause**.

People in withdrawal are often in pain or feeling quite ill. They're also frightened or irritable and very much focused on getting more drugs or alcohol, sometimes by any means necessary. The signs of withdrawal can include:

- **Unstable coordination.** Try to get the person to sit or lie down for their safety.
- **Restlessness and agitation.** Try to reduce any stimulating input.
- **Unpredictable and sudden actions.** Keep your movements calm and slow.
- **Slurred or incoherent speech.** Speak to them in a calm, quiet voice and make an extra effort to understand what they're saying.
- **Disorientation** Provide short explanations of what is going on.
- **Abnormally rigid muscles.** They may present with tense muscles.
- **Being argumentative and demanding.** Try to redirect them or de-escalate depending on the mode of anger or rage they exhibit.

Of course, these behaviors can be symptoms of a number of other syndromes. De-escalation is necessary, however, in order to ascertain what is causing the behavior, and therefore, what treatment is in order.

> **Figure 23.2 Calming of patients in withdrawal**
> Be calm and firm. Redirect them when they get very demanding. Reassure them and use appropriate de-escalation strategies so that you can calm them enough to render medical assessment and treatment.
>
> There is no specific withdrawal rage. They will display terrified, chaotic, hot, cold, or predatory rage (Section IX). Use the tactics that best fit the mode of rage they're experiencing.

CHAPTER 24

Psychosis—Delusions and Hallucinations

Whatever the diagnosis (i.e., schizophrenia, schizoaffective disorder, bipolar disorder, post traumatic stress disorder, depression, drug induced), the syndrome of psychosis is typified by delusions and/or hallucinations. A **delusion** is first and foremost a disturbance in cognition. It is a belief that doesn't fit reality—sort of. A **hallucination** is an unreal perception through any of the senses.

What Is a Delusion?

A delusion is usually referred to as a belief that doesn't conform to reality. Actually, it's a lot more than that:

- People from different cultures may have very different beliefs. Shared cultural beliefs, however, aren't delusional, even if you can't conceive how others could see the world as they do.
- There is often nothing remarkable about the delusional belief except that it isn't true. For example, everyone knows the FBI follows people—the question is if the FBI is following this particular person?
- Lots of people have eccentric beliefs: unconventional religious rites, non-traditional dietary and health habits, or a belief in aliens, crop circles, or telepathy. Some of these may be *your* beliefs; they're eccentric to others, but not to you. Unusual ideas and beliefs, however, aren't delusional.

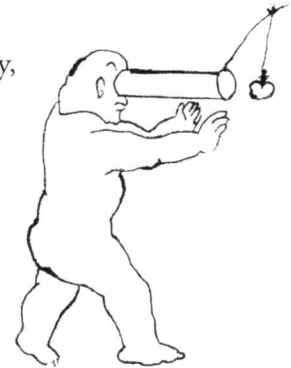

A delusion is like being a member of a one-person cult. All the confusing thoughts the person may have had, all their worries, prayers, fantasies, or ideas suddenly coalesce into **THE BELIEF** that explains everything. Such beliefs are unshakable, inarguable, and unaltered by conflicting evidence.

Types of Delusions

- **Grandiose.** People with this type of delusion believe that they have been appointed to a special mission, that they have extraordinary or unusual powers, or are special, remarkable beings.
- **Religious.** Often linked with grandiose delusions, a patient may become preoccupied with religion, focusing all their attention on their beliefs, which may be self-made or associated with mainstream doctrines.
- **Jealous.** A person may believe, against all evidence, that their partner is unfaithful to them. Jealous delusions surpass the almost always irrational nature of ordinary jealousy. The jealous delusional person concocts infidelity out of the slightest glance, a change in clothing, or a five-

minute delay in returning home, etc. Those who have severe borderline personality disorder, where whatever emotion they feel becomes their reality, sometimes manifest this type of delusional psychosis in periods of stress.

- **Delusional stalking (erotomania).** A person may believe that another person is in love with them, is married to them, or has been somehow designated as theirs, whether they know it or not. (Special requirements for communicating with those who display erotomaniac stalking behaviors will be discussed below).
- **Persecutory (paranoia).** A paranoid delusional person may believe that people, institutions, or other powers have hostile intentions toward them or have committing evil actions against them. They often believe that others are sending energy toward them, thinking about them, talking about them, or looking at them with malevolent intent. In addition to general strategies for managing any psychotic person, there are specific strategies for communicating with a paranoid person (Chapter 19).

What Are Hallucinations?

Hallucinations are perceptions through any of the five senses that don't conform to reality. Hallucinations are often, but not always, accompanied by delusions.

Figure 24 Not all hallucinations are psychotic

It is possible to perceive a hallucination, but be neither delusional nor psychotic. A person may hallucinate, but either has no belief about it, or realizes that it is a disturbance of perception, rather than reality. For example, people suffering from several days of jet-lag may complain of hearing voices. However, they're quite aware that the voices are caused by sleep-deprivation, paying them no more heed than people do when they have a song 'stuck' in their head.

Types of Hallucinations

The following is a list of the different types of hallucinations:

- **Auditory.** There are two levels of hallucinations perceived through hearing. The first level is ***auditory distortion***. One mishears what is said, something that is frequently part of persecutory delusions. For example, a paranoid person is sitting near someone in a restaurant who says, "Do you want the chicken or the ribs?" They hear, "Let's get this chicken in the ribs." The second level is true ***auditory hallucinations***. Close your eyes when someone speaks to you. Do you still hear their voice? Of course you do. When people have auditory hallucinations, the voices are equally real—they are experienced, not merely imagined. That is why you can't simply say, "The voice isn't real,"—that makes as much sense to them as someone saying that your foot isn't real.

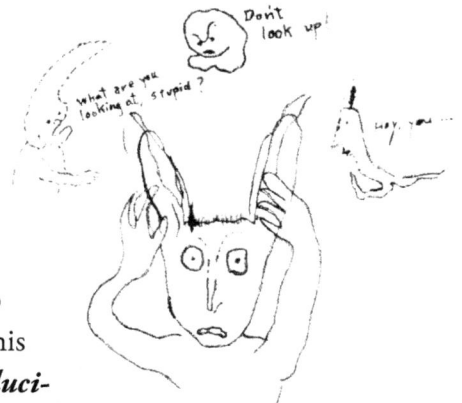

Paranoid people, in particular, often display a 'listening attitude.' They enter a situation that evokes their paranoia, and expect to be victimized, accused, talked about or assaulted. Then they either mishear people based on what they expect to hear, or in more severe cases, they actually hear hallucinatory voices uttering just what they expected or feared.[13]

- **Visual.** There are two levels where people may experience ***visual distortions***. The distorted visual image appears to move, melt, emerge toward them, or even speak. Think of a Salvador Dali painting in which the objects melt and flow. The second level is true visual hallucinations, in which objects or beings appear that no one else can see.

- **Olfactory.** This is sometimes a result or symptom of brain injury, as the part of the brain that detects odors is at the front of the head, a frequent target of injury. If a previously non-psychotic person complains of hallucinatory smells, they need an immediate neurological assessment. This may be an emergent situation that, if not addressed, can result in permanent brain damage. Other people, without head injuries and purely psychotic, can get focused on their own body smells, and believe, for example, that they're rotting away. Other times, they believe they can smell poison gas seeping through the walls.

- **Tactile.** These are sensations felt within the body. The sensation of bugs crawling on or under the skin is a frequent side effect of such drugs as methamphetamine or cocaine. It can also be a manifestation of alcohol-induced delirium tremens. Something very similar to tactile hallucinations can be a side effect of a person's psychiatric medication. Tactile hallucinations are incredibly irritating. Remember the last time you had 'prickly heat,' or some other miserable rash. Remember what it did to your disposition. Now multiply it tenfold. Therefore, always be prepared for anger or even rage on the part of a person who is experiencing tactile hallucinations, even apart from the concern you would always have regarding someone abusing large quantities of meth, alcohol or cocaine.

The Torment of Hallucinations

Hallucinations torment their victims in a variety of ways:

- For unknown reasons, hallucinated voices are almost always cruel. People may be ordered to do awful or degrading things, or they may simply hear disgusting sounds and ugly demeaning words. Visual hallucinations can be as haunting as ghosts. Olfactory hallucinations are often foul, and tactile hallucinations are almost always very unpleasant sensations.

- A person tries to tell others what they perceive, but their experience is denied over and over again. They may be teased or laughed at. Ironically, the people they speak to about their perceptions often torment them in ways similar to the torment of the hallucinations.

- Psychotic patients find that their worldview is called into question every day. They don't know what is real and what is not. Imagine reaching to pick up your coffee, and not knowing if the liquid will disappear from the cup, or if the handle will suddenly twine around your finger like a little snake. Imagine this is true of every object in your life. In such circumstances, people with psychotic disorders find it difficult to trust anything at all.

CHAPTER 25

Communication With Someone Who Is
Experiencing Delusions Or Hallucinations

Disengage

It can be very draining to talk with a psychotic patient. Like a cultist trying to convert you to their group, they may try to convince you that what they believe is real. They may insist that you accept their beliefs, or even more problematic, insist that you *do* believe, but simply won't admit it. They become focused on debating your resistance, or furious that you deny what is, to them, absolutely true.

There is often no good reason to continue such a discussion. Delusions aren't like some sort of backed-up fluid that you vent and drain away. The more the delusional person talks about it, the more preoccupied he/she becomes, and more agitated as well. While delusional people may feel locked in their inner world and desperate to communicate what they're experiencing, discussion and argument seem to cement the delusions even further.

Figure 25.1 Rule #1: Disengage

There are many occasions when nothing at all can be accomplished by talking about delusions or hallucinations. There is no emergency, and no need for information gathering either. In such cases, disengage.

Islands of Sanity

Imagine being dropped overboard into the ocean. It is cold and rough among the waves, and there are all sorts of sea-life that demand your attention: everything from sharks to jellyfish. There seems to be no way to escape, and it is so overwhelming that you can't take your mind off it.

Even in the ocean, however, there are small patches of land: islands. If you can only get to them, you can put your feet down on solid ground. For psychotic people, too, there are 'islands of sanity,' areas of their lives where they aren't delusional. They may be convinced, for example, that someone is poisoning their food, and only canned goods are safe to eat; or that someone is beaming messages directly into their brain. But when you bring up the subject of football, and the two of you begin talking about how the Steelers destroyed the Seahawks yet again, the psychotic person takes his mind off his delusions without even realizing it. For a brief moment, they have a moment of respite—an island of sanity.

Remember, you and other firefighter and EMTs may deal with the same, profoundly psychotic person on a frequent basis. If you have a means of deflecting them out of their delusional rut and into discussing something where they can feel solid, they will begin to associate firefighters and EMTs as beings who stabilize rather than stress them. This, alone, is a significant factor in risk reduction. Therefore, try to ensure that other firefighters and EMTs are aware of what the particular island of sanity is for a potentially dangerous psychotic person.

Figure 25.2 Rule #2: Move towards an island of sanity

Pay attention to where the psychotic patient is not delusional—when they talk about subjects that are not distorted by their pathological cognitions. Whenever they are delusional, try to divert them away from their delusions to those 'islands of sanity.' If the patient gets stuck within his/ her delusions, you may find that changing the subject requires real finesse. Nonetheless, do so whenever you can, because talking about delusions makes it worse.

These islands of sanity are not necessarily 'nice' subjects. One of the authors worked with a very dangerous man for nine months and the only subjects that he wasn't floridly psychotic were bar fights and motorcycles. It was safer talking about the sound of a cue ball impacting on someone's skull than what he had for dinner or what his childhood was like.

WARNING-DO NOT 'LIGHT THEM UP': One person's island of sanity may be funny-sounding, eccentric, or perhaps, at variance with your own beliefs or interests. (For example, they love a football team that you hate). No one on your crew should ever tease or provoke the individual about that island of sanity. Aside from the lack of human decency that entails, you will undermine the safety of all your crew. If the person now associates firefighters and EMS with people who deride something they believe to be special, you will no longer have something stable or sane to shift their thoughts towards when they become agitated or delusional.

Threat Assessment: When should you talk about delusions or hallucinations?

Some of most dangerous mentally ill people are those whom you see over and over again. They frequently decompensate, or go off their medications; therefore, it is necessary to do a brief threat assessment every time you see them.

Imagine a delusional person who is sure that she is the Archangel Michael. If you recall this biblical story, Michael, the righteous sword of the Lord, casts Satan out of Heaven. Further imagine that this woman believes she perceives Satan's work in the behavior of people around her. Based on her past history, you must be aware when she gets preoccupied with her delusions, because some time ago, seeing evidence of Satan's corruption among fire service, she tried to stab one of the EMTs.

Therefore, whenever this woman begins to talk about God, angels, Satan, or anything similar, it is a good idea to ask questions about that which she is preoccupied. Some questions you could ask her follow:

- Mrs. Hampton, are you telling me that you think you have seen Satan? Where?
- Why do you think that this is Satan's work?
- Do you think you should do anything about this?
- What do you think you should do?

If Mrs. Hampton's answers are bland and not aggressive, then carry on with your work. If her answers seem to manifest dangerous ideation, then you must act to get her help, protecting society in the process. For example, if she says, "Don't call me Mrs. Hampton! I'm Michael, the Lord's most beloved angel. Satan will have no place in your hearts when I cut him out!" In such an event, do what is necessary to ensure she is not a threat now (tactical retreat by your crew, call law enforcement, etc.), and get her evaluated by a professional. She may need to have her medications adjusted, or must stay in the hospital for a brief or extended period of time.

Figure 25.3 Rule #3: Talk about the delusions for threat assessment

Do talk about the patient's delusions long enough to ascertain if they are dangerous. If so, get necessary help to ensure safety. If not, change the subject

---

Don't Agree: At Least Most of the Time

It might seem to be easiest to take the line of least resistance—simply agree with the delusions, or pretend that you, too, perceive the hallucinations rather than get caught in arguments with a mentally ill person about reality. There are a number of problems in doing so, however:

- When you agree with delusions and/or hallucinations, you will entrench them deeper into the person's belief system.
- When you agree with delusions or hallucinations, *you* can be incorporated into the delusional system. This can become toxic. You become a necessary part of their delusions, and they begin to stalk you. In other cases, you make a 'misstep.' For example, they believe that you, an emissary of God, have invited them to rule the Earth. However, when you don't deliver on what they believe is your promise, they turn on you in rage, suddenly realizing that you were, in fact, an agent of Hell sent to stop them from ascending to their throne.
- It can be dangerous in other ways. Just because one is mentally ill doesn't mean the person is gullible or stupid. Some street-wise mentally ill people soon realize that you don't really believe in their delusional world. They see you as scamming them or making fun of them. You can create someone focused on you as an enemy.

> ### Figure 25.4 Rule #4: Don't agree with the delusions
>
> In almost all circumstances, don't agree with the delusions. At most, passively accept their perception in the interest of their complying with something that will keep everyone safer.
>
> For example: The ill person states that you are a wise man from a planet from Arcturus. Accepting the 'charisma,' but not the role, you say, "I don't know anything about other stars or planets, but I do want you to get on this gurney now and lie quietly."
>
> The patient replies, "OK, wise man from another star. I'll do what you say."

Don't Disagree—At Least Most of the Time

Common sense seems to demand that you speak for reality. When people see something that isn't there, shouldn't you tell them so? If they have an irrational belief, why not argue them out of it, or at least, diplomatically point out where they're wrong. When you argue with delusional or hallucinating people, however, you're telling them that their perceptions are lying to them. It is unlikely that telling them that the world as they see it isn't real will improve that rapport.

Sometimes, however, delusional people may ask, even plead with you, for disagreement because they don't want to believe what their delusions seem to tell them. At other times, a hallucinating person can make a tenuous distinction between real perceptions and hallucinations and will ask if you think something hallucinated is real. In these cases, *when you have been invited*, it is acceptable to state that not only do you not perceive the hallucination or believe the delusion, but also that you don't think they are real.

> ### Figure 25.5 Rule #5: Don't disagree—at least most of the time
>
> Don't engage in arguments about whether the psychotic person's perceptions are real. However, if they ask you for a 'reality check,' then you can state that you don't believe that the delusional belief is correct or the hallucination is real. In this case, you are helping the person understand that what he/she perceives is not the 'rule' of the world.

An Important Exception to the "Don't Disagree" Rule: Delusional Stalking

All stalkers should be viewed as potentially quite dangerous.[14] They have an absolutely selfish, entitled sense of their own right to approach or harass the victim, either in person, or as is becoming more common, through the use of electronic media such as text messages, email, or social networking websites. **This is a crime, and the victim needs to be protected. Law enforcement should be contacted in all cases where you encounter a stalker.**

A small subset of stalkers is neither obsessed nor trying to regain control of a relationship they have lost. They're delusional. They truly believe that the object of their interest is married to them, destined for them, or that there is some absolute condition that justifies their pursuit. If you are interacting with such an individual, you must directly say that it isn't true that the victim is destined for, in love with, or otherwise involved with them. Don't get into long discussions, much less arguments. Simply state that it isn't true. Anything less than complete contradiction will be taken as agreement by the stalker.

Figure 25.6 Rule #6: Exception—disagree with the delusion of erotomania
Calmly and directly tell the delusional person they have no right stalk the victim. Refuse to discuss it further, attend to your professional responsibilities and contact law enforcement.

Differentiation: Distinguish Between Your World and Theirs

Delusional beliefs are nearly inescapable. When people experiencing psychotic symptoms attempt to discuss their delusions with others, they're often brushed off, minimized, or even ridiculed. Of course, firefighters and EMTs should never act so callously or dismissively, although as we just learned, you can neither agree nor disagree with them either. Can you do anything to get the mentally ill person to recognize the distinction between your world and theirs, so that you aren't merely part of their psychotic world? **Differentiate** yourself from them.

Simply stated, to differentiate is to perceive or express a difference. As used in this context, the authors mean that the firefighter or EMT should acknowledge the person's perceptions and beliefs. At the same time, while informing them that although you don't share their perceptions, you aren't arguing that theirs are invalid, unrealistic, or fantastical. You are, however, encouraging the psychotic person to concede that other viewpoints do exist. Here are some examples:

- Alice, I see the table and chairs, the pictures on the wall, and the books on the floor, just like you do. But you see something that I don't. I don't see a vat of boiling oil in the corner of the room. No, I'm not saying you don't see it. I believe you do. I'm just saying that it's something you see that I don't. I don't know why, but that's the way it is.
- Sal, I only hear two voices in this room—yours and mine. I don't hear a woman's voice at all. What do you hear her say?
- Jamey, I know about the democrats and the republicans. I've never heard of the Illuminated Ones. I'm not arguing with you here. I'm just saying that I've never heard of them, so I'm not the person to talk about them.

Remember, the point here isn't to convince them that their delusions aren't real, or even that they're wrong. Essentially, differentiation helps you keep the lines of communication open while not getting sucked in to their perspective. Think of two people from different cultures, trying to explain what it is like to live in their respective worlds, or even two beings from different planets. If the mentally ill person finds himself/herself shut-down or discounted when they try to talk about their perceptions or beliefs, it is likely that they will try to shut you down in return.

In some circumstances, you can act in concert with their belief without endorsing it. For example, "I can't see the laser beams, but I know lasers don't pass through solid objects. Maybe you will feel safer sitting in that ambulance over there."[15]

Figure 25.7 Rule #7: Differentiate

Give the patient the 'right' to their own perceptions and beliefs. Inform them that you don't perceive what they do, but you aren't arguing with them about what *they* see or believe. In some cases, take their delusions into account without agreeing with them. Example: "I don't see any razor blades on the tree branches, but if I did, I wouldn't walk around in the park after dark where I couldn't see what I might run into. I'd stay home when the sun went down."

Steam Valve: When the Pressure is Too Great

Some people, either psychotic or manic (Chapter 26) are so full of things to say, think or feel, that they seem like they're going to explode. Their speech can become pressured as well. Words burst out of them in a cascade.

- Sometimes they make sense, but they totally dominate the 'air time' in the room, talking over other people. Even if there is a task to be done, they can't focus and they make it nearly impossible for you to focus as well.
- Other times, they make no sense whatsoever. Their words may sound like poetry as they link words by sound, not by meaning.
- They may jump from idea to idea, in what are called 'loose associations,' or 'tangential thinking.'

With some such people, you sometimes have to take over, saying, "You have talked enough for awhile. It's time to be quiet." This sometimes works quite well for both sides. It is honest, it is direct, and it sets a limit. At other times, however, one needs to let out a little pressure like opening a valve in a steam pipe. *Then* you take over, saying one portion of what you have to say.

- Let them speak until you get the theme of what they are saying.
- First, put out a hand, palm down, fingers curved at waist level to interrupt them. If they don't perceive it, put up both hands, using a little drama in your facial expression to get their attention and interrupt.
- In letting them speak for a little while about their preoccupations, you've let out a little pressure, so to speak.
- Sum up what they said in a sentence or two. Use a little energy in your voice to prove that you're really 'with' them. Then, ask or say something, getting either some compliance or a bit of information. For example: "That is serious. Politics right now are terrible! You HAVE to tell me more about this left-wing conspiracy, but before you do, how many pills did you take?"

- In exchange for this information, let them return to their cascade of ideas, allowing a little more pressure to be released.
- Then, once again, firmly interrupt, sum up, and require something else.

In essence, you sum up what they said to prove you were listening, and *then* ask your question or make your statement. Steam-valving is for the purpose of letting the person tell enough of what is pressuring them internally so that they don't fight you for the conversational floor.

Figure 25.8 Example of steam-valving

Larry (Patient). "And then the Berlin Wall came tumbling down and the spirits of dead communist babies flew over the rubble…."

Firefighter/EMT. "Larry. Wait. I want you to tell me more about those communist babies, but before you do, did you swallow some pills?"

Larry. "Yes, I had to take medicine to save myself, and dead communist babies have flown into the ears of all the children of the West and that is why they no longer respect their elders or money or eider down pillows, or…."

Firefighter/EMT. "Larry, I'm worried about the children too! Kids ARE different these days. I want to hear more, but first—what pills did you take?"

Larry. "The blue and green pills, the one's that say to sleep forever, and never wake up, and…."

Figure 25.9 Rule #8: Steam-valving

This is useful with people whose speech is a cascade of words and ideas that are either all over the place (zigzag) or delusional. Listen and then interrupt. Sum up what they said, and tell them you want to hear more, but before they do, you have a question (or instruction) for them. Then let them return to their cascade of words. Listen a bit more, then interrupt again. Continue with multiple sequences of release of pressure, interruptions and questions until you get the information you need.

Physical Space, Physical Contact, and the Use of the Eyes with Psychotic People

Concerns about eye contact and physical contact are incredibly important in regard to people with psychosis.

- Even more than in ordinary circumstances, be acutely aware when you're inadvertently 'pressuring' the psychotic person by standing or sitting too close to them. Consider this *your* responsibility—don't expect the psychotic person to necessarily tell you. The first sign that you're too close—**if you aren't paying attention**—may be an attack, as the psychotic person believes they must protect themselves from your 'invasion.'
- Other psychotic patients aren't aware whatsoever of personal space, and stand or sit too close to you. Firmly, without aggression or heat, tell them to move back. "Monty, I really want to hear what you're saying. But you're standing too close to me. Step four steps back and tell me more."

- For many psychotic folks, direct, sustained eye contact seems to pierce them to the brain. It's as if you can read their thoughts. Other mentally ill people can misinterpret direct eye contact as aggressive, threatening, or seductive. Therefore, if they're uncomfortable with being directly looked at (you'll know it!), occasionally 'touch base' by making brief eye contact, then ease your eyes away, and then back again. Of course, **never take your eyes off of the person in a manner that would make you unaware of any precursors to assault.**

Figure 25.10 Rule #9: Body Spacing, Body Contact, and Eye Contact

Be aware of physical spacing—don't stand too close, and don't accept the person standing too close to you. Most psychotic patients are made anxious by direct eye contact, experiencing it as either a threat or a challenge. Limit eye contact when it is not emergent so that you have to establish control through command presence, a situation where direct eye contact is a necessity.

CHAPTER 26

Tactics For Dealing With
Symptoms Of Mania

Mania is a state of high energy. People in this condition need little sleep, and can be excited, grandiose, agitated, or irritable. They often have flights of fancy, which can be either creative or completely irrational. Their speech is often pressured. Not only is it rapid, but also there is a sense that there is more to say than they can possibly get out.

They're usually extremely confident, even to the degree of believing themselves to be invulnerable. Manic people are often narcissistic. They feel wonderful, and their own needs and desires are the only things that matter. Their judgment can be extremely poor and they engage in behaviors that can put them or others at risk.

The manic state is associated most commonly with bipolar disorder (manic-depression), in which periods of mania are one-half of a cycle in which the other is periods of depression. **Some drugs can also cause manic episodes (particularly stimulant drugs such as amphetamine or cocaine), and not infrequently, mania can also be a side effect of psychiatric medications.**

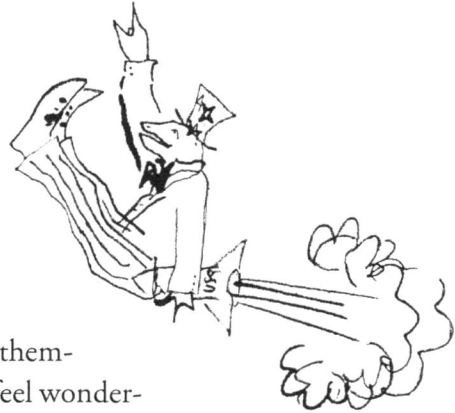

Figure 26.1 Extreme Manic State

People with different brain malfunctions can have periods of agitation that may look very much like mania, but this kind of delirium is usually more extreme than the classic manic state. Such patients are usually quite confused and disorganized. On the other hand, manic people can get so agitated, called "manic excitement," that they shift into a delirium state. All such patients, whatever the cause, are de-escalated using the strategies described in Chapter 49 on Chaotic Rage.

Manic people are particularly vulnerable because they're most in danger when they feel wonderful. Imagine the best spring day of your life. The sky is blue, birds are singing, and a gentle breeze keeps things just cool enough to be comfortable. You wake up and literally jump out of bed, happy to be alive. You have so much energy that it feels like there is champagne in your veins. Imagine that feeling day-after-day, multiplied ten or twenty times. Can you see how easy it would be to begin to make unwise choices, how your confidence could lead you to, for example, hijack that freight train because you always wanted to be an engineer?[16]

When you feel this good, it seems like a good idea to feel *even better*. Thus, manic people often want to party. Drugs and alcohol are very tempting, spending money to buy anything and everything you want leads to credit cards run to the max, and often the energy turns sexual and the manic person gets involved with people who may be inappropriate for them or even dangerous. On the flip side, manic people—stimulant drug users or not—sometimes try to calm themselves with other drugs: barbiturates, heroin, and alcohol. Alcohol can have a 'paradoxical effect' on some manic patients, further exciting rather than sedating them.[17]

Manic people often talk in rapid cascades of words, a waterfall of ideas leaping from one area to another. Sometimes you can follow their thoughts, although they're speaking very rapidly, but at other times, they verbally zigzag, making connections that have little or no meaning. In extreme manic states, people can become psychotic, with all the symptoms of grandiosity, persecutory, paranoid, and religious delusions that any other psychotic patient might have.

Some manic people become very irritable. They can have a hair-trigger temper, and may also be provocative. Rather than merely being reactive, some will aggressively tease and taunt other people. It may seem to be in good fun, at first, but it goes too far—way too far. Others may simply try to pick a fight.

Brittle Grandiosity

Manic people can act as if they don't have a care in the world. They spin ideas, one after another, and expect both agreement and admiration. They seem utterly self-confident. However, truly self-confident people are resilient; unfair criticisms seem to bounce off them. Think of manic grandiosity, however, as a fragile structure, like a tower of spun sugar. It glitters, it glows, and it's huge! But tap the wrong strut or beam and the entire tower falls down in shards. For example, if you directly criticize patients who are manic, they can experience your criticism as a personal attack, and from giddy happiness, they suddenly turn on you in rage. If you tease them about their somewhat irrational ideas, try to joke around with them, or laugh at something funny that they said, they easily misinterpret this, too, as an attack, thinking you're making fun of them.

In other words, consider the manic flight of words to be a kind of hysteria. Even when they appear happy, it is as if they're on a giddy flight hanging onto a helium balloon. It certainly is thrilling—until they look down! Miscalculated teasing or criticism is experienced as if you're poking at the balloon with a needle.

Figure 26.2 One Author's Experience: Be Careful—All Is Not What It Seems!

WARNING: They may be acting like comedians, but they aren't trying to be funny!

One of the writers recalls a little guy who had lined up over five thousand 'matchbox' cars on every projecting surface of the inside of his house. None were glued, but they were perfectly balanced, even onto the molding on the walls! Because he had overdosed, we took him to the hospital. He was given charcoal, and as he sat on a gurney, belching black fluid down his chin into a pan, he was talking non-stop, chirping like a little bird, asking why, if this medicine was so bad, they had given it to a man like him? He suggested Skittles™ instead. It was both a reasonable question and under the particular circumstances, funny. One of the nurses began to laugh, and he slung the metal basin he was holding right at her head, and still spewing black vomit, grabbed her by the throat, screaming, "This isn't funny. Nothing's funny!"

Watch Out! Mania Can be Infectious

Being with manic people can be very exciting, particularly if they're at low or moderate levels of elevation. They can be brilliant conversationalists—witty, sexy, provocative, and entertaining. They're fast on their feet, bawdy, and full of fun. It is easy to catch the mood of someone like this, easy to begin to feel grandiose and over-confident yourself. Getting swept up in this energy is just as dangerous as it would be on the highway—once you've jumped in the back seat and are zigzagging down the road at 90 miles an hour, it's pretty hard to get back out of the vehicle.

Many manic people assume, when you 'hitch a ride,' that you're in absolute agreement with them. They assume that what they want is what you want. However, when you object, they can suddenly turn on you in ferocious, betrayed anger. There is an old expression: "He's a drag," referring to someone who slows the party down. That isn't a bad idea with the manic person. Therefore do the following:
- Stay centered.
- Don't get swept away.
- Focus on slowing things down. Speak slower, and take things step-by-step.

It is possible to use humor in a tactical way with manic persons. But you need to be calm and centered (Section II). If you have 'caught' the manic contagion, and are trying to match wits with them, the funny statement you make will backfire on you. **Your purpose must be to catch their attention and slow things down, not have fun with them.**

Medication and Bipolar Disorder: It's Not Like Diabetes

Bipolar patients have a unique problem: medication can usually control their symptoms, but they're most ill when they feel wonderful. Perhaps they will be calm, more organized, sleep more hours, and not get in trouble if they take their medications, but life will lose a wonderful glow. Unlike almost any other condition, profoundly 'ill' manic patients often feel right with themselves: in a state of mystic transport, ecstasy, or just plain fun. People with bipolar illness won't take medication unless their lives on medication are rich and interesting, so much so that they're willing to spurn the dangerous wonders that the manic state seems to offer. For the bipolar person, going *off* their medications is the equivalent of the drug addict using again.

Once off their medications, folks with bipolar disorder can crash down into severe depression, leading to an apocalyptic attitude that there is no hope that things will ever get better: suicidal ideation or rage toward others can easily follow. Even more dangerous, they may quickly amp up into a manic episode that can combine grandiosity, elevated mood, high energy, poor judgment, irritability and psychosis. As a young woman with bipolar disorder, who also had affection for methamphetamine in large doses stated, "The difference between meth and mania? Well, mania is MUCH bigger. Huge!"

When encouraging a bipolar person to take medications, many professionals and family members say, "It's a condition like diabetes. You need to take it every day to maintain yourself. It's not like medicine for a sore throat that you take until you're cured, and then never have to take again." This is true, but there is a very profound difference between diabetes and bipolar disorder. If you don't take your medicine for diabetes, you very quickly become seriously ill. If people with bipolar illness discontinue medication, very often they will feel much better than when they were on the medications. Unfortunately, all too often, that puts them and many others at risk.

Boisterousness—"Nobody Gets Hurt in TuneTown"

Manic people sometimes get loud and provocative, laughing and playing around. On the surface, this boisterousness seems happy—and happy people aren't dangerous, are they? However, this boisterousness is actually a kind of aggressive buoyancy. There is an 'edge' to it, like a bully in a bar who insists that you engage in a drinking contest, or hugs you until your ribs crack. Remember the phrase in the movie Roger Rabbit—"No one gets hurt in TuneTown." Boisterousness, particularly when displayed by a mentally ill or intoxicated person lacks all sense of proportion. The person does whatever they feel like, without any concern that you might be injured.

Figure 26.3 Review: Dealing with a patient in a manic state

You will recognize the manic person because they will display super high energy. They will often be talking very fast and their ideas will "zigzag" from one to another. They often act like comedians, with a rapid-fire delivery. Their behavior may also be either sexualized or hair-trigger aggressive. In either case, they will very likely be provocative. Here are some things you should do:

- Remain calm and centered.
- Be conscious of their "brittle" state of mind, in spite of how confidently they behave. Grandiose doesn't mean strong!
- Don't bluntly criticize their actions.
- If you use any humor, it is for the purpose of slowing them down, not joking around.
- Don't join in what sounds like fun. It isn't.
- They may try to provoke you (think of the Road Runner and Coyote).
- They can be very volatile, exploding into rage with the slightest provocation. Be relaxed but ready for the worst.
- Boisterousness is not fun or friendly—it is a potential precursor to assault. Try to de-escalate and calm them, but be prepared for that apparent happiness to suddenly shift into something very dangerous.
- If the manic person is also psychotic, the latter will probably take precedence. In these situations, you essentially have a hallucinating or delusional person who also happens to be moving and talking very fast.
- If the manic person is in full rant, cascading words in an unending stream, use Steam Valving (Chapter 25—Rule #8).

CHAPTER 27

Communication With
Elderly People

Effectively dealing with elderly people, particularly if they're also mentally disabled, can be one of the most challenging situations that a firefighter or EMT might face. Firefighters and EMTs will almost always outweigh and outmuscle the elderly person who, even if they have retained substantial strength, may be physically fragile and need to be managed with care.

Are there any verbal interventions that might possibly keep the situation under control at a lower level of force with an elderly, demented patient? Remember, older adults aren't a monolithic category. They're people, just like us, simply older. Everything—every character type, every mode of aggression, every mental syndrome, and every de-escalation strategy—applies to elderly people as well as those of other age groups. Despite their age, elderly people do assault others, particularly those involved in their care. Their rage can emerge from dementia, medical conditions, pain, adverse drug mental illness, pure meanness or hate, or any number of stressors including abuse by their own caregivers.

Be aware that the elderly may be resistant to help. This may be due to disorganization and confusion brought on by dementia, a combination of severe depression and fear, or by pride ("At least I still have the strength to refuse someone"). Another manifestation of pride is self-reliance—an often estimable character trait that, in the case of many medically compromised people, can result in serious conditions being neglected because asking for help is viewed as a personal defeat. The following will be helpful in handling the elderly:

- Speak respectfully, befitting the age and seniority of the person. Too many people speak in a patronizing demeaning tone to elderly people, and even when cognitively impaired, they may know they're being talked to as if they're children.
- Don't forget that they may be hard-of-hearing. What you think is resistance may be due to them not being able to understand or hear what you are saying. This is particularly relevant for women, who tend to speak at a higher register. High frequency tones are usually the first to be unheard as a person becomes hard-of-hearing. An elderly person may be irritable with a female firefighter or EMT, not because they have 'issues' with women, but because they are irritated as they struggle to hear what the higher voiced person is saying.
- Use their honorific and last name unless specifically invited to use their first name. If you wish to achieve a more informal relationship, ask "Would you prefer to be called Mrs. X or by your first name?" Let them *offer* their first name.
- When it is not an immediately emergent situation, take a little bit more time. Attempt to 'nibble around the edges,' talking about life, about family. Sometimes the volatile rage that elderly

people display comes from a deep depression—they're isolated, confused, and no one seems to care if they live or die.

- Be prepared to get enormously frustrated at their leaden stubbornness, as you find that "they simply won't do what is good for them." What appears to be inertia may be a profound expression of fear. Remember that the most proximate change that many old people are concerned with is death, and therefore, any situation provoking anxiety evokes the fear of death. **You may think they're defiant; they may simply be scared out of their wits.**

- Don't talk around or about the person to others as if they aren't present.

- Don't barrage them with choices, decisions, or too much information.

- Paranoia, (Chapter 19) whatever the cause, is one of the frequent triggers of rage in elderly people, particularly with older adults with dementia or adverse drug reactions. As the person becomes suspicious, you can often change the subject, so that the object of their suspicion recedes from their awareness.

- The rage and violence that emerges with elderly people is frequently chaotic. (See Chapter 22 on details regarding communication with disorganized people and Chapter 49 on de-escalation of people in chaotic states).

- Be aware that the person's behavior may very possibly be brought on by improper use of their prescribed medications, or interactions between different prescribed and over-the-counter medications.

Figure 27.1 Concerning physical restraint and the elderly

If you must use physical restraint tactics to safely bring an elderly person under control, be aware of the particular vulnerabilities of elderly people, who are generally quite brittle as well as frail. Ensure that the type of physical guidance and restraint you use offers the least risk of injury. This should be integrated into your training scenarios, and best-practice restrain techniques for the physically frail and vulnerable must be regularly practiced. With a combination of verbal soothing, and the use of several individuals incorporating gentle restraint at the shoulders, hips and knees, an elderly person can be controlled with hands-on pressure. **We cannot underscore this strongly enough— a broken bone, particularly a broken hip, may be a life-threatening injury.**

Elderly people bruise easily and have paper-thin skin. You may cause severe bruising or superficial lacerations if the elderly person is aggressively restrained

The first responder must also be aware of the medical condition of the patient before administering a chemical restraint as they may cause respiratory depression and respiratory arrest. Be prepared to resuscitate the patient if they go into respiratory or cardiac arrest

---

SECTION V

Recognizing The Strategies
Of Opportunistic And
Manipulative Patients

CHAPTER 28

Divide And Confuse—
Borderline Personality Disorder
And Splitting

Figure 28.1 Author's Note
Individuals with borderline traits frequently display suicidal and para-suicidal behaviors. These behaviors will be discussed in detail in **Section VI**.

Personality disorders are habitual patterns of behavior that sometimes cause an individual, and almost always others associated with them, considerable problems. Most types of personality disorders, however, do not cause behaviors that significantly affect safety. Several, however, are often associated with dangerous behavior: paranoid personality (Chapter 19), anti-social personality, with its most intense manifestation, sociopathy (Chapters 29-30), and a third type called borderline personality disorder. An individual with borderline traits believes that whatever feeling they are experiencing right now is their only possible reality. For example, an individual is accidentally bumped in the line at the bank. Instead of brushing it off, he explodes. This is a borderline reaction. On the flip side, he meets his somewhat sympathetic EMT, and within five seconds, he knows that she is the love of his life.

Any of us can be overcome by feelings that seem beyond our control, or make emotional decisions that are not in our own best interest. Falling in love, for example, is often a borderline state. Sometimes we are impulsive, and sometimes we get angry, even enraged. For us, however, such experiences are unusual. For the individual with borderline personality disorder, they are an everyday occurrence.

Those on the mild end of the spectrum will be quite emotional, over-reacting to things that others could take in stride. For those whose disorder is more severe, it is as if their nervous system, at least that part which regulates emotion, seemingly lacks any protective sheathing. Imagine trying to live your daily life with two layers of skin peeled off; this, on an emotional level, is borderline existence. One's current emotions are inescapable. The person with borderline personality traits lives with the intensity and the emotional lack of resilience of a toddler. They experience the world and the people in it as good and bad, perfect and foul. Many are frequently arrested for domestic violence, road rage, and impulsive fights ("What are you looking at!").

Figure 28.2 Examples of people with extreme borderline personality traits

The two main characters in the movie, *Monster*, starring Charlize Theron and Christina Ricci, are portrayals of women with two types of extreme borderline personality disorders. Theron plays Alicia Wournos, a woman who came from a horrendously abusive background, drifted into prostitution, and then murdered six 'johns.' She had the emotional stability of a toddler, shifting from sweetness and trust to hair-trigger rage. Whatever she felt at that moment was her only reality. Some of her murders, at least, were based on the threat and abuse she *felt* she was experiencing from the johns.

The Ricci character was a woman of almost no character at all. She templated to whomever she was with at the time. Rather than a person with an 'active' borderline syndrome, like Wournos, she was passive. Like Wournos, however, all her actions, too, are based on feelings alone, not on any rational evaluation on what was good for her, in this case—bonding with a dominant, violent individual, and then, later, betraying her to her law enforcement interrogators.

Because of this combination of character traits, individuals with borderline personality disorder frequently find themselves in various crises. Among them are genuine suicide attempts and para-suicidal acts (self-mutilating behaviors or repeat suicide 'gestures staged for discovery and attention), all of which to be discussed in detail in Section VI, impulsive acts of assault, and brief psychotic episodes (Chapters 24 & 25).

A firefighter or EMT may discover that other EMTs, police officers, mental health case managers, lawyers, psychologists, and nurses disagree how to respond to the borderline patient, even to the point of arguing about whom is at fault for their current crisis. In particular, those involved in a therapeutic relationship with the patient often lean to 'contextualizing'—explaining, or excusing their behavior, especially when the patient has a previous history of trauma or abuse. When the providers and others associated with an individual displaying borderline traits get tangled up in intense disputes about what is best for them, this type of conflict is called *splitting*.

Splitting doesn't happen in a vacuum. The individual with borderline traits, although not really conscious of what he or she is doing, presents a different facet of their personality to each person with whom they interact. Such behavior is strategic: whether they are aware of it or not, it is a 'divide and confuse' tactic. If people are arguing about you, they can't gang up on you.

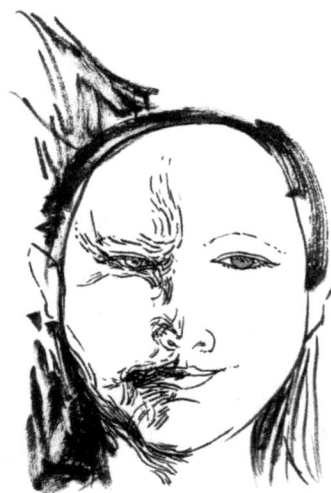

It is not surprising, really, that such a patient will appear quite different to a counselor trying to build a supportive relationship, as opposed to the doctor in an emergency medical facility, who is not happy whatsoever to see the bloody-wristed patient for the tenth time this month, or to the firefighter or EMT who is rescuing them from their latest emergency.

The firefighter or EMT can, of course, make unilateral decisions based on the requirements of an emergency, but if all members of the *de facto* team responsible for such an individual remain at odds, your 'victory' will be short-lived. You will be working with the same people on other cases, and you will most likely continue to work 'at odds together' regarding this patient. Thus, whenever a team gets intensely at odds regarding a single patient, suggest the possibility of splitting, and see if you can, by comparing observations, see if their interactions with various people have created the adversarial situation in which you find yourselves.

Finally, individuals with borderline personality disorder are, not surprisingly, quite reactive to other people's emotional reactions. The attitude of the firefighter or EMT should be someone who wishes the patient well, yet undeviatingly enforces rules and protocols. By maintaining a type of 'warm emotional distance,' you won't get emotionally worked up over things, and the patient will find less to react to as well.

CHAPTER 29

Bad Intentions—Recognizing The Strategies Of Opportunistic And Manipulative Patients

In order to satisfy their need for instant gratification, some patients attempt to manipulate nearly everyone with whom they come into contact. Some use manipulation as a means of furthering criminal actions; while others view people in general as opportunities to gain something they want. A few others live for hate and destruction, and delight most in duping people so that they don't even know how 'dirty they were done' Some manipulative individuals lie so that no one can pin them down, using a 'divide and disappear' strategy so that the more powerful beings in their life argue about them, instead of focusing directly on what they are really doing.

Manipulative Strategies

Manipulative strategies can result from a variety of emotions and intentions, such as those born of revenge, malice, desperation, laziness, guilt, or as the result of drug and alcohol use.[18] (NOTE: All of the following descriptions may apply not only to patients, but also to collateral contacts such as family and friends). You must be vigilant in detecting manipulative behaviors, and require proper verification of any information given by the patient. Paradoxically, you should be wary of patients who appear to be overly compliant, especially those who have committed serious offenses, such as sex crimes or offenses involving the use of weapons or violence. Quite often, some of the most dangerous individuals will be the ones who are, apparently, low-risk patients, complying with any requirements in their current setting. This seemingly compliant behavior may in fact be nothing more than an attempt to manipulate and control *your* behavior. What the manipulative patient is likely trying to accomplish is to create conditions so that you do not see what they are up to. After all, why would you focus much attention on a truly compliant patient!

Some manipulative patients use stories to overload you with information to keep your attention away from what they are doing. They try to charm you so that you actually look forward to contact with them, yet remaining unaware of what is really going on.

Manipulative patients will also ask you for personal information, such as marital status, children, in which part of town you reside, and so forth. These questions seem to be innocent enough, just the normal back and forth of a conversation. What the manipulative patient is doing, however, is gathering information, something that they can use later in the relationship, or perhaps use to fuel their current fantasies. Firefighters and EMTs should refrain from answering any personal questions a patient may ask, and redirect any conversation back toward your professional duties.

Manipulative patients are also quite adept at behavioral observations, such as noting the body language of others. They are particularly interested in potential victims, those who are easily intimidated or frightened, including other patients. They are also interested in those who put up any kind of a front, including an attempt to appear tough. All the manipulative patient has to do is challenge them, and the 'fronting' firefighter or EMT begins reacting like a yo-yo on a string, trying to keep up appearances, to someone who has already read them inside and out.

Manipulative patients are also likely to blame others for both their failures and their behaviors. Nothing is ever their fault: they were simply in the wrong place at the wrong time; they didn't know they left the pills on the table where their child could find them, and anyway, it's the doctor's fault for not 'warning me good enough' how dangerous they were.

Manipulative patients view their relationships as transactions, with an eye toward gaining an advantage or placing other individuals in their debt. Firefighters and EMTs should always be wary and always be thinking about what a patient has to gain from any interaction. One major type of relationship manipulation is that of flirtation and sexuality, which can manifest in any gender configuration. You must address any flirtatious behaviors or sexual innuendo with the patient immediately, and follow through with appropriate written documentation. While this may be embarrassing, it is the only way you can let your administration know, formally, that the patient's behavior was addressed and boundaries were enforced. If this issue is not addressed instantly, the patient will view it as implied acceptance on your part. It may also lead others, both patients and co-workers, to assume that something is going on. By following through with written documentation, this allows the firefighter or EMTs supervisor to take further action if the patient's behavior continues. This is yet another of the many reasons that firefighters and EMTs should not be isolated while interviewing patients, regardless of gender.

CHAPTER 30

Tactical And Safety Considerations
Related To The Sociopathic Patient

Figure 30.1 Sociopaths stand alone

There is considerable overlap in this chapter with the safety recommendations made throughout this book, particularly in the chapter on manipulative behavior (Chapter 29). In Section IX, we will discuss what to do when facing someone presenting with Hot, Predatory, or Aggressive-Manipulative Rage—all modes that the sociopath can manifest. In this chapter, the authors will highlight the most salient point's specific to sociopathic individuals. We believe that this information is so important to firefighter and EMT safety that it must be presented as a stand-alone chapter for easy reference.

Psychopath and sociopath are largely inter-changeable terms. The former, in fact, has once again been incorporated into the lexicon of psychiatry after a hiatus, where it was largely abandoned. However, far too many people get confused between psychosis and psychopathy, even though the former, a disturbance of cognition and perception is far apart from the latter, a disturbance of morality. Therefore, we will use the term sociopath, so there is no possible confusion.

The term sociopath evokes very strong reactions. Estimates are that 1-3 percent of any population, and perhaps 40 percent of any jail population is sociopathic. A small percentage of individuals commit most of the crimes in any society, and although there is a sociological component to crime, the sociopath, to a remarkable degree, seems independent of such factors.

The entertainment media, as well as sensationalized news accounts of horrendously violent killers and rapists, has introduced an image of the malevolent criminal mastermind or the sadistic predator into the public's consciousness. Without a doubt, violent sociopaths do exist, but even so, they are often rather mundane in appearance and affect, blending in with their surroundings without attracting any undue attention.

Figure 30.2 Examples of sociopaths in the movies

Instead of thinking of some movie monster such as Hannibal Lector, a much more useful image would be Johnny Depp's character in *Pirates of the Caribbean*. In his role as Captain Jack Sparrow, Depp plays an aggressive narcissist; he is attractive and likeable, but also utterly selfish and quite willing to violate social norms. A second image would be the Matt Damon character in *The Talented Mr. Ripley*, an inoffensive chameleon-like man, who has no particular desire to kill anyone, but when circumstances 'require' it, he does so without hesitation.

Although sociopathic patients can be charming and ingratiating, they can also be violent, provocative, dishonest, arrogant, and quite willing to break any rule. Some are remarkably talented, even brilliantly creative. They are aggressive narcissists—the only thing they really care about is themselves. Everything we have just discussed in regards to manipulative strategies in the last chapter is relevant to a discussion of sociopathic patients. However, the sociopathic patient presents problems beyond what you will experience with the 'ordinary' criminal personality, however manipulative the latter may be. Not only do they lack a sense of remorse at the harm inflicted upon their victims, they often take delight in it.

Just as a leopard or a cougar is known to attack whenever a vulnerable animal turns its back and exposes its neck, sociopathic patients feed off vulnerability. Because of their manipulative charm, they can easily get under the defenses of others. They will gravitate to the most vulnerable people on your team. They study everyone with whom they come into contact, making note of any apparent weaknesses and developing new strategies of manipulation and control. For example, "Hmm, when EMT Gibbs tilts her head and smiles while I'm talking, I find myself relaxing a little. I can use this the next time I'm trying to get close to that girl I saw in Ward D. I've got to get hospitalized again!"

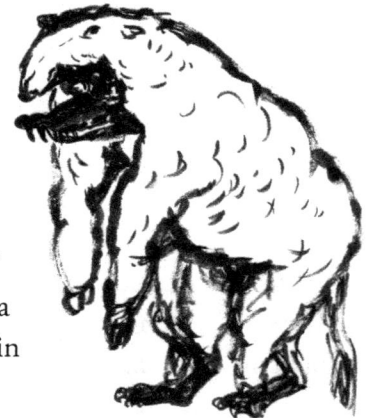

Without a doubt, the most dangerous are the sexually violent sociopaths, who use their guile to groom others for exploitation, prior to enacting sexual assaults. Although common sense would dictate against a firefighter or EMT ever fostering a personal relationship with any patient, it does happen. A sociopathic patient may attempt to groom and seduce a firefighter or EMT, just for the thrill of destroying their career, or for the purposes of blackmail or privilege. Such patients owe their allegiance to no one, although they may form quasi-sentimental attachments that last until a stronger interest or desire pushes them away. This loyalty is on the level of, "Who do you think you are, patting my dog without my permission!"

Sociopaths are often impulsive, and their sense of invincibility often leads them to ignore consequences. Their impulsivity can also result in sudden and unexpected displays of violent behavior if they don't get what they want. Many sociopaths, however, are 'instrumentally violent,' using it as a tool: 'just business,' so to speak. For others, the act itself is gratifying; they are sadistically violent. In sum, sociopaths propensity for physical and emotional violence, coupled with their charming manipulativeness and the fact that there are **NO** therapeutic interventions that can 'cure' them, means you must remain observant and wary at all times when dealing with them.

When interacting with such a patient, firefighters and EMTs need to remain conscious of the fact that they are quite skilled in reading other people: how strong they are, their susceptibility to manipulation, and most significantly, what danger they represent to the patient. Quite simply, they are out to destroy you by one means or another. The authors recommend strongly Robert Hare's illuminating work, **Without Conscience: The Disturbing World of the Psychopath** for a detailed discussion of this subgroup of patients.[19]

Figure 30.3 Substance abusers may present as sociopathic

Substance abusers often act like psychopaths while actively using. Addicts in remission who truly are engaged in treatment usually begin to abandon manipulative and strategic behaviors. Sociopaths, on the other hand, don't. They may use different strategies when they are sober, but they will never abandon a tactical, manipulative approach.

Tactical and Safety Considerations

The following is a list of tactical and safety considerations for EMTs and firefighters.

1. **You will be attacked through your 'best' and your 'worst' points**. Of course, the sociopathic patient will attack your weak points. If you are insecure about your personal appearance; for example, the sociopath will either make you feel more insecure, or in a more sophisticated tactic, reassure you that he or she, at least, finds you quite attractive. What is harder to notice is when you are attacked through your best points. For example, if you appear to be physically fit, they will try to consult with you about your exercise regimen, or ask where and when you workout. If you love children, they will find a way to ask your advice on an alleged phone call from their ex-wife about putting their child on medications. They might really have a child who needs medication. But they are asking you in order to gain some traction, not to get your help. For such an individual, anything can be leverage. Remember, they don't even have to lie. The truth is an even better tool!

2. **Notice when others start making excuses for the patient.** When conned or manipulated, people often find a way to rationalize what the sociopath is doing, or has done. For example, after a near assault on an EMT who responded to his overdose, a counselor says, "You have to understand. He was brought up in a hellish environment. When you approached, he 'flashbacked' to the way his father treated him." Don't allow others to suggest that you make any allowances or otherwise undermine your safety based on how *they* 'contextualize' the patient's behavior.

3. **Track any manipulative strategies, document them well, and alert all other members of your team to the manipulative strategies a patient is using.** Consult and consult again. Don't discount the observations of other first responders or professionals. They are often very important, especially those who interact most directly with then patient in question. Consult yet again.

4. **You may be intimidated.** The most obvious manifestation of intimidation is fear. <u>There is always a reason for fear.</u> If you are frightened of any patient, consult with both your own crew and with police. What is more difficult to recognize is an unconscious attempt to avoid being frightened by giving in to the demands of the sociopath! Ironically, the intimidated first responder may sometimes claim that they have a special rapport or working relationship with the patient; when in fact, all they are doing is giving the predator exactly what he wants.

5. **Be aware of grooming behaviors.** The 'grooming cycle' is a pattern of behavior designed to alleviate the intended victim's fears and apprehensions, all the while targeting them for attack. The patient will make their target feel a little off-balance, making them anxious, scared, or flattered. Then they lessen the pressure while making a request that firefighter or EMT would have granted anyway. The patient begins to 'train' you to experience a sense of relief when granting a request.

Figure 30.4 Grooming

The father of a patient stands too close to you (only slightly—not enough to require you to issue a command that they back up). Then, simultaneous to moving back to a more comfortable distance, he asks it would be OK to take notes on your suggestions. His goal is to cause you to associate granting a request with a release of tension. Hard eye-contact, shifting to friendliness, is another common grooming tactic.

If successful, the sociopath will make requests that get closer and closer to a moral or ethical line. Once he can get you to do something *over* the line, however, slightly, you are now compromised: an object of blackmail or worse. Once you start bending the rules, breaking them isn't so far off.

6. **Guard all personal information.** As discussed previously, personal information can be used in a variety of ways. The sociopath can use such information to determine points of leverage against you. They can talk publicly about you, apparently displaying intimate knowledge of your affairs. In the worst case, such information can be used to track you down outside of your professional life, or make you fear for the safety of your friends and family.

7. **Don't get beyond the horizon line.** <u>Don't meet sociopaths alone!</u> You are vulnerable to manipulation when no one is present to witness and monitor the interaction with the patient. You may not even perceive manipulation is happening. Remember you are vulnerable to physical attack at any time the sociopathic patient believes that it is to their advantage, if their rage is triggered, or simply because it would be enjoyable!

8. **Detecting calculated splitting.** As stated earlier, the sociopathic patient uses gossip, rumors, misdirection, and blatant lying to set all the stakeholders involved in their supervision and treatment against each other. Regular communication and consultation with the various members of the treatment team is the best way to detect and confront splitting.

SECTION VI

Suicidal Individuals

CHAPTER 31

EMT And Firefighters' Role
In Response To Suicide

Suicide is an apocalyptic action—literally self-annihilation. For the suicidal person, however, it is an attempt to solve a problem. They find themselves in an intolerable situation, and nothing makes their pain any less.

First responders aren't counselors. Therefore, one could legitimately state that suicide should be the responsibility of a mental health professional. Nonetheless, mental health issue that it is, and problem-solving activity that it might be, suicide is also the killing of a human being. That it is done by one's own hand doesn't make it less murderous. This is a particularly important consideration because, given that there is hatred and often a weapon involved, you must consider the safety of others who might have any connection—even mere proximity—with the suicidal person. In short, the difference between murder and suicide is often no more than what direction the weapon is pointing.

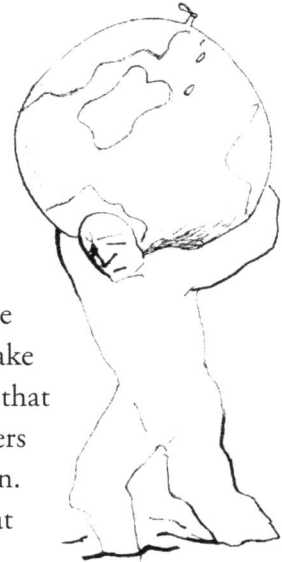

Firefighters and EMTs voice a lot of concern about 'suicide by cop,' dangerous behaviors that are enacted to force a police officer to do the 'job' for the suicidal person. This concern is justified—far too many violent encounters with police are 'victim precipitated.' In other words, an individual does something deliberately to get a police officer to kill them. One great way to get a police officer to shoot oneself is to threaten or actually harm anyone nearby—in this case, you.

This is not your greatest risk, however. Just as more police officers die by their own hand each year than all line-of-duty deaths (including homicide, accidental deaths and illnesses related to the job),[20] fire services are seeing an uptick in firefighter suicides as well. The suicide assessment that you do may be to assist a brother or sister on your crew who is in terrible personal trouble—depressed, distraught, traumatized, or otherwise in such pain that *they're* considering suicide. If no one has the courage to ask, they will remain alone with their pain.

Warning Signs

What should make you consider the possibility or even likelihood that someone might be suicidal beyond them bluntly stating that fact? Below are some warning signs:
- Significant negative changes in the individual's life: divorce or a romantic break-up, events such as fights at school or the workplace, an incident that is humiliating, a large disappointment such

as being dropped from a team or club in the case of youth, or fired in the case of an adult, etc. Personal losses aren't only of social position or status: due to a deterioration of one's physical or emotional health, it may have become difficult, if not impossible, to do the things one used to do. Consider, therefore, firefighter and EMT injuries, that may make it impossible to do the job which defines a man or woman as who they are.

- Warning signs that suggest such negative psychological changes even when you don't have concrete information: a radical change in clothing or appearance, particularly styles that sets one apart from the society of which they were previously a member, a lack of care about one's appearance, hostility towards peers, crewmates, or family, social withdrawal, social isolation, giving away prize possessions, writing or drawings with morbid or despairing themes, a depressed demeanor, allusions to a lack of a future or to the 'pointlessness of it all,' or paradoxically, reassuring statements when you know nothing has changed for the better, such as "You don't have to worry about me anymore. I'll be taking care of things. It's not an issue, anymore," etc.

- Sometimes, without knowing why, you have a sense of foreboding, or at other times, one thinks something 'ridiculous,' like, "I don't think that kid will live to see 20," or "I wonder if this is the last time I will see this person." Such thoughts are often, let us emphasize, <u>very often</u> an intuitive sense that something is wrong. Asking someone if they're suicidal when your 'evidence' is so vague requires some tact, but approach you must.

- Statistically, suicide is the tenth leading cause of death for adults in the United States and third for adolescents.[21] It is important to note that 3-5 percent of those who are suicidal don't seek any help and successfully kill themselves; in addition 30 percent leave it to chance whether someone intervenes; on the other hand, 65 percent don't wish to really end their lives. Eight out of ten suicidal individuals give some form of warning as to their intent. Hopelessness, helplessness, and not seeing a solution to their problem(s) are the hallmarks of a suicidal individual.

CHAPTER 32

The Basics of Intervention With Someone You Believe Might Be Suicidal

Are you the proper person to ask this individual any questions at all? This isn't the place for grandiosity, where you believe that because you're 'good with people,' that this person will open up to you. Do you *know* that this person respects you? If not, you're probably not the person to speak with them. To be sure, there are people who are isolated and alienated, and it is *only* through the asking of the questions of concern that respect between you will be born. But you must at least have a sense, knowing this person, that he/she doesn't hold you in either personal contempt or indifference. If you become aware that you can't establish any rapport or mutual respect, then you need to pass this task on to another firefighter or EMT.

To underscore again, the suicidal person may not be a patient at all. Firefighting and EMT work is enormously stressful, both on you and on your family. Every once in a while, someone hits a breaking point. If no one asks the questions that need to be asked, they may end up killing themselves.

If however, you're the person who has to speak with the suicidal person, what must you do? (NOTE: Some of the following strategies may seem contradictory. As you read them, however, you will be able to imagine or recall the type of person to whom you should approach in that specific way).

Figure 32 Why are YOU talking to the suicidal individual?

Don't assume that this task will be that of a law enforcement officer (crisis negotiator or not) or a counselor. Particularly in rural environments, you may be first on scene. Also, remember again; you may be speaking to someone on your crew, not necessarily a patient.

- **Concentrate and get them to concentrate on you.** You won't get to choose where you engage the individual: a bridge, hotel room, roof top, from outside their car, in a park, etc. The environment may be loud or otherwise distracting. Onlookers may be yelling at the person to jump from the bridge or shoot himself/herself. Use circular breathing to simultaneously give the person close, attention while remaining aware of your surroundings—where your team is and what potential threats are nearby. Whenever the person becomes distracted, get them to focus on you.
- **Demeanor.** Too much direct eye-contact, close physical proximity, or an overly-gentle, 'concerned' voice may shut them down. Speak easily but not over-confidently. If you present yourself as too 'together,' they may experience this as a slap in the face, their lack of ease contrasting

negatively with you. If all you do is stare in their eyes, they will experience it as a constant, intrusive examination.

- **Meander.** With a reticent or wary individual, your conversation should 'wander around,' talking about this and that. As long as they're talking, they aren't killing themselves. This gives you time and also helps to build trust.

- **Ask direct questions.** When you have a real concern that an individual is considering or planning suicide, you must be more direct. Don't tiptoe around the subject, as vague statements leave the person an 'out.' The following would be an example of this mistake with the individual's inner thoughts place in parentheses:

  a. **Firefighter/EMT.** "Are you thinking of hurting yourself?"

  b. **Patient.** "No, I'm not." *(Soon I'll be feeling no pain.)*

  The correct question to ask when a true concern about suicide arises is, **"Are you thinking of killing yourself?" or "Do you intend to kill yourself?"** Being asked questions directly is a relief because it indicates that you are someone who is strong enough to listen to what is really going on inside them. If the person is not suicidal, they will let you know. They should be able to give you a clear explanation why you don't need to be concerned. If they're outraged, explain why you were concerned. One final point: It *won't* put the idea in their head if it wasn't there to begin with.

- **Speak in a calm matter-of-fact tone of voice.** If you sound nervous, you'll appear unreliable. If you're joking or off-hand, the person will feel that you aren't taking them seriously. If you're overly concerned, overly warm, or 'sensitive,' you'll sound like a hovering counselor, that soft-voice, earth-tone wearing, gentle soul who can't be trusted to stand up and fight, but seeks refuge only in being 'nice.' A calm, matter-of-fact tone shows that you aren't panicked by their situation, and that you can handle anything they say.

- **Act as if you have all the time you need.** If you act like there is little time, the person you're talking with will believe you, and they'll rush to a decision or conclusion. When you take time, you give time. The suicidal person begins to believe that there is enough time to figure out a better solution than suicide.

- **Don't give advice too soon.** Until you know the situation, don't hand out advice. Even then, keep it to a minimum. If you immediately say, "Think of your family," the individual might mentally reply, "Yeah, they'll be sorry. Their tears dropping on my grave are the best payback I can think of!"

- **Never dare them to do it.** That kind of stupidity only works in the movies. The classic stupid sentence is, "Cutting? If you were serious, you would cut your wrists lengthwise, not cross-wise." The idea here is to 'scare the person straight.' The aggressive intervener thinks that the patient is obviously attention seeking and not serious, so they try to shock them with the 'reality' of what they're doing. In all cases we can recall, such 'interventions' are born out of frustration, irritation, burn-out, or plain dislike of the repeatedly suicidal person. It is a statement for us, not them. One of the authors met a man who took such advice regarding lengthwise cuts. His crippled arm looks like corduroy, due to seven elbow-to-wrist razor slashes.

- **Don't get in a debate, particularly a religious debate.** Some people use suicidal behavior as a way to feel some power in a world over which they have little control. Debates about the meaning of life, the nature of heaven, or the immorality of suicide will break rapport, particularly if you're 'winning.'
- **The most powerful intervention with suicidal individuals is that you're talking**. The suicidal person, almost invariably, feels completely isolated, cut off from life and from people. A respectful conversation conveys on an almost primal level that they're still worth something because you find them worth talking and listening. Communication itself heals.

CHAPTER 33

Essential Questions Concerning Suicide

> **Figure 33 The last person to see the suicidal person is often viewed as responsible for their death**
>
> Your jurisdiction may have hard and fast rules on what firefighters or EMT should do when contacting a suicidal individual. For example, you may be required to take them to an emergency room as soon as you ascertain that they're suicidal. In other jurisdictions, particularly when there is coordination with the mental health system, some of the responses below will result in the person being linked up with a 'next day appointment' or a mental health outreach team that may appear at the scene of this emergency. **Do not** leave someone alone if there is a possibility they may take their own life. At minimum, 'hand them off' to police or mental health providers. Documentation of the interaction is very important for the patient and for all who will subsequently deal with the person (or review the case later). Remember, the last person to have seen the suicidal person alive is the first person deemed responsible if they later kill themselves.

The following are the standard questions for assessing suicide risk. As you can see, there is a progression in which greater specificity indicates greater danger. You're assessing if the individual is safe, and if not, your next step would be to get them to a mental health professional, or get them placed in custody, depending on the level of risk.

Don't use the following questions as a "checklist." Instead use them in the natural flow of the conversation, in a calm, matter-of-fact tone, while understanding that the individual may wander off on all sorts of tangents before being ready to answer the next question.

The Four Questions

1. **"Are you planning to kill yourself?"**
   - **"No."** If they answer no, follow up with questions and statements why you believe they might. If they can't satisfactorily counter your suspicions ("Your boyfriend called and stated that you told him that you were going out in a blaze of glory tonight. And then you said, 'Don't look for the body.'"), regard this the same as if they admitted to suicidal ideation.
   - **"I don't want to kill myself, but I pray I just won't wake up in the morning."** This could be termed passive or soft suicidal ideation. Don't minimize this. The person's pain is very real. At

the same time, these individuals can usually be linked with a mental health intervention, such as an outreach worker or an appointment the next day.

- **"I'm not telling you."** Try to get them hospitalized if you have collateral evidence that they might be suicidal, so that they can be linked up with proper personnel for a full assessment. It shouldn't be your job to beg them for an honest answer. If you have enough collateral information to suggest that they might be suicidal, you can insist that the proper authorities (police or mental health professionals) assess them for involuntary hospitalization, despite their refusal to answer any of your questions
- **"Yes I am."** <u>Clear red flag</u>

2. "How would you do it?"

- **"I don't know."** This, too, usually means you have time. You should be able to negotiate an agreement to seek or accept treatment after further discussion. You have to find out if there are any impediments to seeking treatment, such as "I'm not going to see a counselor. All they do is look at you and repeat what you say," or the ever more common, "I don't have money to pay for counseling."
- **"I'm not telling you!"** Same as above.
- **"I could do it all sorts of ways."** (They then give you a list in a rather defiant or bored tone.) This is game-playing. It doesn't mean they won't make a suicide attempt, but it usually comes more from an "I'll show you!" attitude than a genuine desire to die. At this point, you must make it clear to them that such suicidal threats are taken seriously. (Depending on the overall situation, the response can range from hospitalization to possible prosecution for false reporting.)
- **A clear method.** "Yeah, I'm going to cut my wrists. I'll be sitting in a bath of warm water, and I'm hoping I'll just drift off." <u>Second red flag</u>.
- **Method and back-up plan.** "I've thought of jumping off the Aurora Bridge, but if I don't have the guts, I'll use pills." Same as above, <u>Second red flag</u>.

3. "Do you have the means to do it?" such as "Do you have a gun." Or "I don't see a car. How are you going to get to the Golden Gate Bridge?"

- **"No, I don't."** Once again, that gives us some time. Despite the serious nature of the first 2 red flags, you may be able to negotiate with them, following up with treatment, or the dispatch of a mental health outreach team. In other cases ("I don't have any pills, but the pharmacy is half a block away and I've got money in my pocket."), you must try to get them detained for treatment.
- **"Yes."** If they're talking about guns or knives, immediately find out if they have the weapon, or where it is located. Alert law enforcement officer(s) and emergency response personnel of the potential threat. In many cases, where the individual is hostile, or in any other way arouses concern within you: <u>clear the scene</u>
- **"I'm not telling you."** Same as above.

4. "When will you do it?" This question helps you gauge immediacy, how established the plan is and if there is anyone else who is "timed" to suffer. (e.g., "On my mom's birthday")

The more "positive" answers you get to these four questions, the greater the risk of a lethal outcome.

Follow-up Questions

In most cases, particularly when interviewing a patient in the field, you will have fully accomplished all that you need to do. You know that the person is or isn't suicidal, and how close to the act they are. In many cases, however, you may have to keep talking:

- They're struggling, yet they trust you, and want to talk more.
- They're on a phone, and you're trying to keep them on the line.
- It is a barricade situation, and the person is talking on the other side of a door.
- They are a fellow firefighter or EMT and you, as a friend, are trying to help them and convince them to seek services.

The following questions are designed to get more information and to keep them talking. As people continue to talk, they often pull back from the intent to kill themselves on their own, or they'll be more amenable to de-escalation because they feel that at last, someone is willing to listen to them. Simple communication brings people away from suicide, even without a solution to the problems that drive a person towards it.

- **Have you tried to kill yourself before?**
- **Have you ever tried to kill yourself another way?** Desperate people become very concrete and literal, thinking only of their chosen method. They may have made several attempts before, by other means.
- **Have you ever *felt* like killing yourself before?**
- **What stopped you? Who stopped you?** Be sure not to make them feel like they 'failed' when they weren't successful in a previous attempt. When they recall someone or something that stopped them, this may help them regain a sense of responsibility for the people who care for them, or some other factor that kept them alive in the past.
- **"Has anybody in your family or someone you cared about ever tried to kill themselves?"** Such people have 'shown the way,' making it seem almost reasonable to the survivors.
- **"Have you been drinking? Using any drugs?"** Don't push this one if you have a sense that the person will be more worried about getting arrested for use or possession than finding a solution to the situation.
- **"What's happened that things are so bad that suicide makes sense?"** OR **"What happened TODAY that you decided to kill yourself?"**
- **"What else did you tried to do to get yourself out of this situation?"** (Be careful—a prickly person could respond by thinking or saying, "OH, SO YOU THINK I'M STUPID." Or "NOW I HAVE TO EXPLAIN MYSELF AGAIN—I DON'T **KNOW** WHY HAVING A GIRLFRIEND AND STRAIGHT A'S ISN'T ENOUGH!!!!!!!"
- Other areas to talk about include if the individual has suffered any recent losses, is ill, or has little or no social/family support.

CHAPTER 34

The Art Of Communication With The Suicidal Person

The following will be helpful in communicating with the suicidal person:

- **Dialogue is the lifeline.** Suicidal people feel profoundly alone. They believe that nothing can end their pain, but death. They're often depressed or very bitter and angry. When one is isolated, one doesn't even feel half-alive, because to be human is to be in relationship with others. When you're able to begin a dialogue with the suicidal person, beyond anything you say, the power resides in the fact that you're speaking together. By definition, the person is no longer alone. Someone is hearing them out. Someone grasps, or at least listens to how terrible life is for them. As time passes, the very fact of talking with you makes them feel alive again, and this gives hope, even when the person's situation has otherwise not changed.

- **Don't make guarantees of how wonderful life will be or how easy it is to recover from one's pain.** When the suicidal person makes demands of you, don't give a guarantee of results. Explain the difficulties instead. For example, "No, I'm not guaranteeing counseling will help. And you will have to work to find a *good* counselor. Even then, it won't be easy. It might be the hardest thing you've ever done. But it's something you haven't tried." Or, "From what you say, that clearly wasn't the right counselor for you. There's better out there. It won't be easy—you'll have to interview them and make sure they are suitable."

- **Do not 'bait and switch'** – Never lie to the patient to get them into the ambulance. Even if you succeed in doing this, they will never trust a first responder again, and future incidents, which happen all too often with many such individuals, will consequently be much more dangerous.

- **Be very careful about making promises about what will or won't occur if they end a standoff situation.** For example, you say, "I promise you will be able to see your child at the hospital once you come down." Later you find out that his wife has a court injunction against him seeing the child, as part of their bitter divorce battle. Once trust is destroyed, the person will be more at risk and less trustful of getting some help next time.

- **Don't be a cheerleader.** If you're too active, too 'positive,' it is as if you're saying that you are 'in it together.' Their success will be your success. Paradoxically, if you act as if things are *too* important, the suicidal person begins to feel that they're doing things for you, not for themselves.

- **Don't try to bolster their 'self esteem.'** You may know that they've got a talent, that they're attractive, or have a wonderful family. The problem is that they know these things too, and it doesn't help whatsoever. If you point this out to them—"You have so many reasons to live!"— you will most likely break rapport entirely. They look in the mirror and they see the beautiful face, but inside, they feel corrupt and foul. They look at their mom and dad, whom they painfully and deeply love, and think, "They would be so happy without me." They have a talent, and they know it, but even as they play the piano or paint or score 30 points in a game, they merely feel an aching misery.

Figure 34.1 Deepening Rapport With the Suicidal Person

Once you have achieved a deeper level of rapport, it is quite sound to talk about what the person loves: their vocation, hopes, and dreams, their family, or their talents. The goal here is to participate in reminding the person of the value of their life. However, they have to realize this, themselves as they talk about these things. It isn't effective to tell them what is special about them. If that were all it took, they wouldn't be suicidal in the first place.

- **Frame things with negatives.** "You've had a bad time. There is no doubt about that. Yet, somehow, you held it together all these months. What's different about today?"
- **Identify the intended 'victims.'** Try to ascertain whom the suicide is intended to hurt. You will be able, thus, to get a better sense if the person is also homicidal, or on the cusp between self-harm and an intention to take others along. We can tell if there are others intended to suffer when we ask:
  a. "Who will find your body?"
  b. "Who will identify your body?"
  Some people are utterly shocked at these questions, so preoccupied with their own pain that they didn't even think that their children, for example, who would be the one to find them upon returning home from work. Others describe that same scene with happiness—hoping thereby that their family member will never have a good night's sleep again.
- **When you should talk about their family.** A natural follow-up of the last question is to begin speaking about their family and what will be the implications of their suicide upon them. You must be careful here. The suicidal person may become enraged with you, perceiving this as a manipulative trick to make them feel guilty. However, once you get a sense that the suicidal person does care for his/her family, particularly children, such talk may be very powerful. For example, one intervener asked a man on a bridge what he would say to his daughter were she the one standing on the railing. As he began to think and speak about this, the intervener was able to suggest that she would probably want to say the same thing to him.
- **Suicide is selfish.** If you get a sense that they do love their children, partner, or friends, but are so preoccupied by their own pain that they don't realize the implications of their suicide on others, one can ask, "What happens to your pain if you do kill yourself." Quite frequently, the suicidal person says that their pain will be over. The reply to that, in a regretful tone, is, "That's not really true. You just wrap your pain up in a package and hand it to your loved ones to carry." This can sometimes shock the person to considering the implications of what they're doing. **Caution:** This type of intervention only comes after some long talking. Many suicidal people are so

focused with their own situation that they become too preoccupied with their own pain to care about their family. Rather than a healthy shock, they will resent you for reminding them of what they're trying to extinguish.

- **Suicidal threats without following through are not a betrayal of *you*.** You will deal with people who dramatize their problems, only later to minimize or discount those who gather to help them. Particularly with people who make repeated attempts or threats, this can enrage or frustrate us. It is ironic that contempt, irritation, or frustration is exactly what they expect from people, and that is what their behavior elicits. One of the occupational hazards of working with people who suffer is that not all those in pain are endearing. Some are frankly quite unlikeable. Others don't even have the ability or resources to accept help when it is offered. It is the hallmark of a professional that you don't become burned out simply because some people either play games, or are playing on an entirely different field than you thought.

How to respond to internal questions that sidetrack us:

- **"I don't know if I would want to live in such a miserable situation."** It's not about you! The fact that they're talking with you means they still have some hope for another answer, even if you cannot imagine what it is.
- **"Why is it important that they live?"** OR **"I know I should care, but I don't."** In cases like these, make death itself your enemy. Your attitude should be that you will do your best to speak for life. You're a voice from the land of the living to one trying to cross over into the land of the dead. *Not on your watch!* If they wanted to die, they shouldn't have come into contact with you!

CHAPTER 35

Suicide As Self-murder—
A Taxonomy

Figure 35.1 The concept of 'self-murder'—an evaluation tool

This is a tool that can be used to help gauge the seriousness of the person's suicidal intent, and what type of suicide it might be. Given that suicide is a form of murder—of oneself—let us categorize it by roughly the same sub-divisions that we do homicide. This type of information can help you know what you should be talking about and how to approach the person. Furthermore, it can be invaluable information to pass onto those who will be working with the person next, such as crisis negotiators, emergency room personnel, mental health professionals, and corrections staff.

- **Aggravated first degree self-murder.** This would include killing oneself in a heinous or torturous way: drinking acid or lye, for example, because the person believes he deserves to suffer. Another example would be a suicide calculated so that a loved one will find the body. A third would be a suicide-murder: killing oneself after killing family members or other people.
- **First degree self-murder.** This would include any planned suicide. The majority of the people to whom you speak will fall into this category. That is why the standard assessment questions are concerned with planning.
- **Second degree self-murder.** This includes impulsive actions that are usually due to extreme emotion or intoxication. Precipitants would be something like a sudden business reversal or a break-up of a relationship. One's world has suddenly turned upside down, and the person's impulsive solution is to 'get out.' It is rare that you will be on-scene *during* an event like this, but it could happen, where the person goes into an explosive personal crisis in your presence. For example, you are rendering aid to a woman in front of her family, when law enforcement shows up and presents a warrant for her arrest. She is so humiliated that she ends up on the apartment roof threatening to jump.
- **Self-harm with intent to commit mayhem.** The person doesn't mean necessarily to die, but they do something horrible to themselves, often with the intent to show others, "See how much I'm suffering!" Or "See how much you make me suffer." We're aware that the distinction between the previous item and this one is a hard call. You may not even be able to make it at all. However, if you were aware that the person didn't consciously intend to die, a professional would work with them in a different way. The professionals to whom you might refer such an individual would also find this useful information, if you happen to acquire it.

Figure 35.2 An accidental 'suicide'

One of the authors recalls a case where a young man returned home to find his father on the couch having sex with the young man's new girlfriend. (He was unaware that his girlfriend and his father shared affection for crack cocaine. When she first entered the home, they recognized each other as kindred spirits immediately.) The young man pulled out a fish boning knife and yelling at the two of them, stabbed himself right in the abdomen. Miraculously, the flexible blade threaded its way between his internal organs and all he needed was a few stitches. He said to me, "I didn't want to die. I didn't even think of that. It's just that my dad has always done stuff like that to me. Every time I trust him, this is the result. I guess I didn't know whether to stab him for doing it, or stab me for being so stupid as to trust him again. I didn't want to die. I just didn't know what else to do."

- **Assaultive self-harm.** This includes suicidal gestures, cutting oneself and other self-mutilating actions. (Chapter 36)
- **Self-sacrifice.** Rare though it may be, this would include actions that have the intention of helping others—like throwing oneself on a grenade to save ones comrades.

Figure 35.3 An Example of self-sacrifice

A young girl, age 6, disclosed sexual abuse by her father, and her mother slapped her in the face for "talking dirty." She continued to suffer in silence for years. When she was 11, her father began turning his attention to her younger sister. Her mother had already made it clear to her that disclosing didn't help, so in that magical thinking of a child, she thought that if she did something as awful as suicide, maybe someone would save her sister. Thankfully, her attempt to kill herself failed, and a very good hospital social worker asked the right questions. She revealed the abuse, and both girls were rescued from their parents.

- **Self-execution.** This includes suicide that is primarily directed by a sense of guilt. Such an individual believes that they deserve to die for some unforgivable transgression. In some cases, they are people who have actually done something terrible; in others, they are suffering from a sense of pathological guilt brought on by mental illness, even though they haven't truly done something terrible.
- **Survivor's guilt.** This particular form of 'self-execution' is usually the outcome of a traumatic event. It is particularly common among frontline war veterans. The bonds between warfighters are among the most profound relationships that humans can experience. Facing death, only the trust and dependence upon one's comrades may keep one alive. A powerful sense of being 'of one flesh' develops, where the man on the right is one's right arm and the man on the other side is one's left. When comrades are killed, one can simultaneously feel like a part of oneself

has been killed, but at the same time, one feels terribly guilty to still be alive, as if one has abandoned one's comrades. One feels like one doesn't have the right to the joys of life. They may believe that the other person or people were better than them. Perhaps worst of all, it may seem that life-and-death is a random throw of the dice, which suggests there was no meaning to one's comrades' sacrifices.

- **Mercy self-killing.** This category includes so-called 'assisted suicide' or other suicides in which the person is seriously ill and wishes to 'die with dignity.'

- **"I'm taking my body out of here."** This is an attempt at final control over one's fate, something that can range as an act of heroism against intolerable violation or oppression to the act of a sociopath in prison whose only way of thwarting the people who hold him against his will is to kill himself/herself.

CHAPTER 36

Crying Wolf—Self-mutilation
And Para-suicidal Behavior

One of the most confusing actions that a person can do—at least to those outside the situation—is self-mutilation. When it is more severe, appearing at first to be a suicidal act, it is referred to as 'para-suicidal behavior.' This primarily includes cutting ones wrists or other actions that, taken to an extreme, could have resulted in death. Among self-mutilating actions we have encountered are:

- Rubbing an eraser on the body until all the skin is peeled away and one has weeping lesions in the flesh.
- Stabbing oneself repeatedly by dropping a knife between the fingers, any error resulting in a wound in the web between the fingers.
- Running a needle in–and-out of the flesh of one's belly.
- Burning the face and genitalia with lit cigarettes.
- Cutting or stabbing wrists, inner elbows, arms, genitals, thighs—anywhere a blade could reach.
- Hacking one's wrists on the corner of a table, and then, after being stitched up, tearing out the stitches with one's teeth and attempting to spray blood on nearby correctional officers.
- Literally slicing open the abdominal wall all the way to the fascia that holds the organs.[22]

The hallmark of all of these actions is that the person doesn't intend to die. Even in the last horrifying example, the woman in question called for help after she's made the cut. There are a number of reasons why someone would do such acts:

- **Self-hatred.** The individual punishes himself/herself through self-torture and disfiguration.
- **Attention seeking.** These cases usually are typified by more superficial wounds. Such individuals 'require' others to pay attention to them, particularly family members or loved ones who become afraid that they will be responsible for their death if they don't act. The case, cited above, of the young man who threaded a needle in-and-out of the folds of his belly was an unpopular, socially inept boy who, by means of this action, got some attention from schoolmates.
- **'Primitive medicine.'** Like ordinary Europeans and Americans a mere 150 years ago, they're metaphorically 'draining out' the poison by 'bleeding' themselves.
- **A struggle to feel something.** Some people, in the throes of deep depression or trauma, literally feel numb. The torturous acts help them feel alive.
- **Stress Reduction.** Physical wounding, like many other stresses on the body, result in the release of endorphins, neuro-hormones that are close analogues to opiates such as morphine and heroin. People can become habituated to endorphin release, and activities that stimulate it can become addictive—one cuts to feel a sense of well-being.

Figure 36.1 Stress reduction by self-wounding

A young woman told one of the authors that, after years of verbal and emotional abuse by her father, "I felt like I was walking on egg shells all the time. Then, when my mom and I finally left, it was like I couldn't stand any emotions at all. Even when I was happy, I would still feel like I was going to explode." She described one day cutting herself on the forearm with an Exacto knife, and to her shock, felt a sense of warmth and peace. Not psychological warmth alone, but a warm floating sensation as well. Several weeks later she tried it again, in a short period of time, it became an addiction.

- **Rehearsal.** Some people want to commit suicide, but they also want to live. Over and over again, their feelings at war within, they make hesitant attempts to harm themselves, and fail.

Figure 36.2 The line of self-mutilation has 'moved'

The 'line' of self-mutilation has moved. We see individuals with multiple piercings, including one's tongue or sexual organs, who have voluntarily branded themselves, and others who even have implants of metal placed under the skin, to end up with 'devil's horns.' Most of these people talk about endorphin release. Many claim that they're making their own bodies into works of art. As strange or repulsive as we may find some of these body modifications, this isn't an emergency, unless the person puts themselves at medical risk.

In an ambiguous situation, you need to ascertain if this is a suicide attempt, and also try to determine how seriously they're wounded. If it is just some grotesque body-modification, that would be their prerogative—unless you believe that they're severely mentally ill where, just to be safe, you should get them evaluated by a mental health professional.

In short, action is necessary if you have either a psychiatric emergency (a genuine suicide attempt) or a medical emergency, either intentional or accidental. Imagine a person who had NO intention of suicide, but decided on a do-it-herself splitting her tongue in emulation of a snake (one author has seen such an unlovely sight. It takes a lot of days and a fair amount of dental floss.). That is her right—it is a bizarre type of do-it-yourself cosmetic surgery. However, when you arrive for a field-check, you find that the bleeding isn't stopping and she's toxic with some sort of infection.

Frequent Fliers

Para-suicidal individuals are often extremely high users—and abusers—of the emergency response system. Many of the problems engendered by their behavior are unsolvable. In Western society, we view this as a manifestation of mental illness or emotional desperation, and generally speaking, believe ourselves required to try to help the person. This requires our law enforcement and emergency medical personnel to strive to intervene, repeatedly, in the behaviors of people who either reject our help, or repeat the actions as if all our interventions are irrelevant. Let us consider the damage their actions cause:

- **Compassion burnout.** We get sick of such people. We see them only as manipulative, self-involved pathetic losers. Beyond whatever justification one might find for that point of view, it unfortunately expands. Many first responders begin to view all mentally ill people, particularly all suicidal people, through the distorted lens that burnout creates. One loses compassion. This becomes a safety issue. When we begin to view others with contempt, they may respond with their own negative emotions. Thereafter, interactions between first responders and the mentally ill become increasingly volatile. This puts everyone at risk. Don't forget that the suicidal, perhaps mentally ill, person might have a interaction with one contemptuous firefighter or EMT, and decide to take it out on another, at a later date.

- **Damage to society.** Suicidal threats, alone, can take up an enormous amount of staff-hours, not only for firefighters and EMT, but also for the emergency medical system as a whole. With our economy severely stressed, and our medical system currently in unknown financial waters, the hundreds of thousands of dollars that may be needed, every year, to manage the behavior of a single para-suicidal individual make such acts, however unintentional, an act of violence against our society. The bottom line is that hard-working citizens pay for any public service.

- **First responder out-of-reach.** Although to the best of our knowledge, such research has never been done, it is a fair assumption that, in the hundreds of thousands of hours that first responders spend dealing with para-suicidal individuals, firefighters and EMT have surely been delayed or unavailable to respond to another medical emergency.

When these individuals (sometimes referred to as 'frequent fliers') come to the repeated attention of firefighters or EMT, a care-and-response committee needs to be set up to figure out the best way to deal with the situation. Ideally, this committee should include representatives from law enforcement, emergency medical response, hospital ER, the mental health system, and the prosecutor's office.

- If the person has made repeated suicidal threats without action, and no other effective intervention has been achieved, they should be prosecuted. Among the charges that can be levied are: false reporting, abuse of the 9-1-1 system, or interfering with medical care. While in detention, it is the responsibility of the mental health system to maintain contact with the person, and begin to work with them so that they get a sense of reward when NOT using suicidal threats to get attention. If the reader's response is that it isn't currently practicable in your community, your agency should initiate a coordinated discussion between law enforcement, mental health professionals, emergency medicine and prosecutors/district attorneys to make such action possible in the future.

- If they have actually enacted suicidal gestures, even wrist scratching or taking a few pills, no one will prosecute them.[23] The risks of a more serious suicidal attempt will be viewed as too high. However, a comprehensive plan can be set up so that the individual gets more emotional rewards and attention by NOT engaging in para-suicidal gestures.

Example of a Plan Developed to Assist a Chronically Para-suicidal Individual

Shauna was somewhat developmentally disabled, with borderline personality disorder (Chapter 28). In other words, she was, emotionally, much like a toddler in an adult body. Whatever she felt, she 'became.' She was in a mental health program that used a 'nurturing model.' In other words, the counselors believed that if they were supportive and accepting, Shauna and the other women in the program would do best. For that reason, they "encouraged, but never directed." Among the things they encouraged Shauna to do was to have more of a social life.

Shauna lived in a rough area of town, but following her counselors' suggestions in her own way, she began going out to bars near her apartment. Naïve, childish, insecure, and quite overweight, she was perfect prey for predators. A man would approach her, speak nicely to her, and suggest they go somewhere private. She'd invite him back to her apartment, where she would be raped. In each case, after the attacker left, she would cut her wrists deeply and then call 9-1-1 for help. Even though this happened on a number of occasions, no investigation was successful. She couldn't describe her attacker, except in terms such as, "He was a nice man. He had blonde hair. Why did he do this?"

Because of her childlike nature, most people remained kind. The police talked gently to her as did emergency medical technicians. She was taken to the hospital, where the nurses, doctors, and social workers took care of her, followed by a 'rape victim advocate,' to be followed by a mental health outreach worker. She would have multiple follow-up appointments with her therapist, who comforted and nurtured her.

One day, a coworker and I were discussing the case, and we essentially came to the conclusion that we, in the system, had become part of Shauna's rape cycle. Each time she would go to the bar with high hopes of meeting someone, she would be violated and cut her wrists, *requiring* a number of kind, strong, wise people to care for and comfort her. We couldn't stop her from going out to bars, we couldn't move in with her to stop the rapists, but we could, without violating any ethics, respond differently. Here, in brief, is the plan the team developed:[24]

- **Police response.** Response time and attempt to investigate crime unchanged. However, each officer was to have a flat affect—nearly emotionless, 'just the facts,' approach to their interview with Shauna. They shouldn't be cold, mean, punitive, or sarcastic. Simply take the information.
- **Emergency medical services.** Emergency medical care unchanged. However, there should be no comforting voice or gesture, no matter how much Shauna was crying or wailing. They should move her to the gurney in a matter- of-fact way, like she was a sack of potatoes.
- **Emergency room.** Medical treatment unchanged. Anesthesia, was, of course, used when stitching her wounds. (Despite any imputation to the contrary, we weren't punishing her. We were also not rewarding her.) The doctors and nurses, however, asked no questions beyond what was needed for medical treatment. The social worker, too, would take just the basic facts. If she needed something to drink, she would receive water, not juice or anything sweet. 'Sweet' means nurturance; we didn't want to nurture her into being raped and possibly killing herself, or being killed by her rapist.

- **Rape victim's advocate.** As might be imagined, these big hearted people, doing a job that few of us could handle, had the hardest time with the plan. With sufficient discussion, however, they understood. Their approach was to be 'distantly kind.' In other words, the same kind of approach one uses with a child who skins their knee—you tend to them and send them on their way. If you make a big deal out of it, they will think it is a big deal as well.

- **The emergency evaluator for mental health would do a full evaluation.** If Shauna wasn't immediately suicidal, she was to be sent home. (This, by the way, was always the case. She slashed herself immediately after the sexual assault, as a means to initiate the 'help' portion of her cycle of behavior. She wouldn't do it again in relation to the same incident.)

- **Welfare check.** Shauna would get a call once daily from the crisis line that was kept brief. She would be reminded to see her therapist and the date and time of her next appointment.

- **Counselor's responsibility.** Her counselor, at their meeting, would have Shauna go through everything she did that night in exhaustive detail, including questions as to why she did not call 9-1-1 *before* cutting herself. In a sense, the counselor initiated an 'after-action review,' something that was not emotionally rewarding in the least. On the flip side, once this was complete and better safety planning was done, ("Don't go to bars anymore," for example.) they would talk about other things, and Shauna would get *emotionally rewarded* for non-pathological discussions, thoughts, and actions. The idea was that Shauna would get no emotional reward for suicide or dangerous actions and *much more* reward for healthy behaviors.

Several weeks subsequent to the implementation of this plan, Shauna again made a suicide attempt after a sexual assault. Everyone held to the plan, although some later confessed that they felt like brutes, seeing this child in an adult's body, walked out of the ER, sobbing like her heart was broken. Her counselors began to work with her according to the plan. A month later, it happened again. Then, the plan 'took.' For a period of over 12 years, she had no contact whatsoever with law enforcement or the emergency medical system, nor did she suffer from any more sexual assaults.[25]

SECTION VII

Recognition of Patterns
of Aggression

CHAPTER 37

The Nature Of Aggression

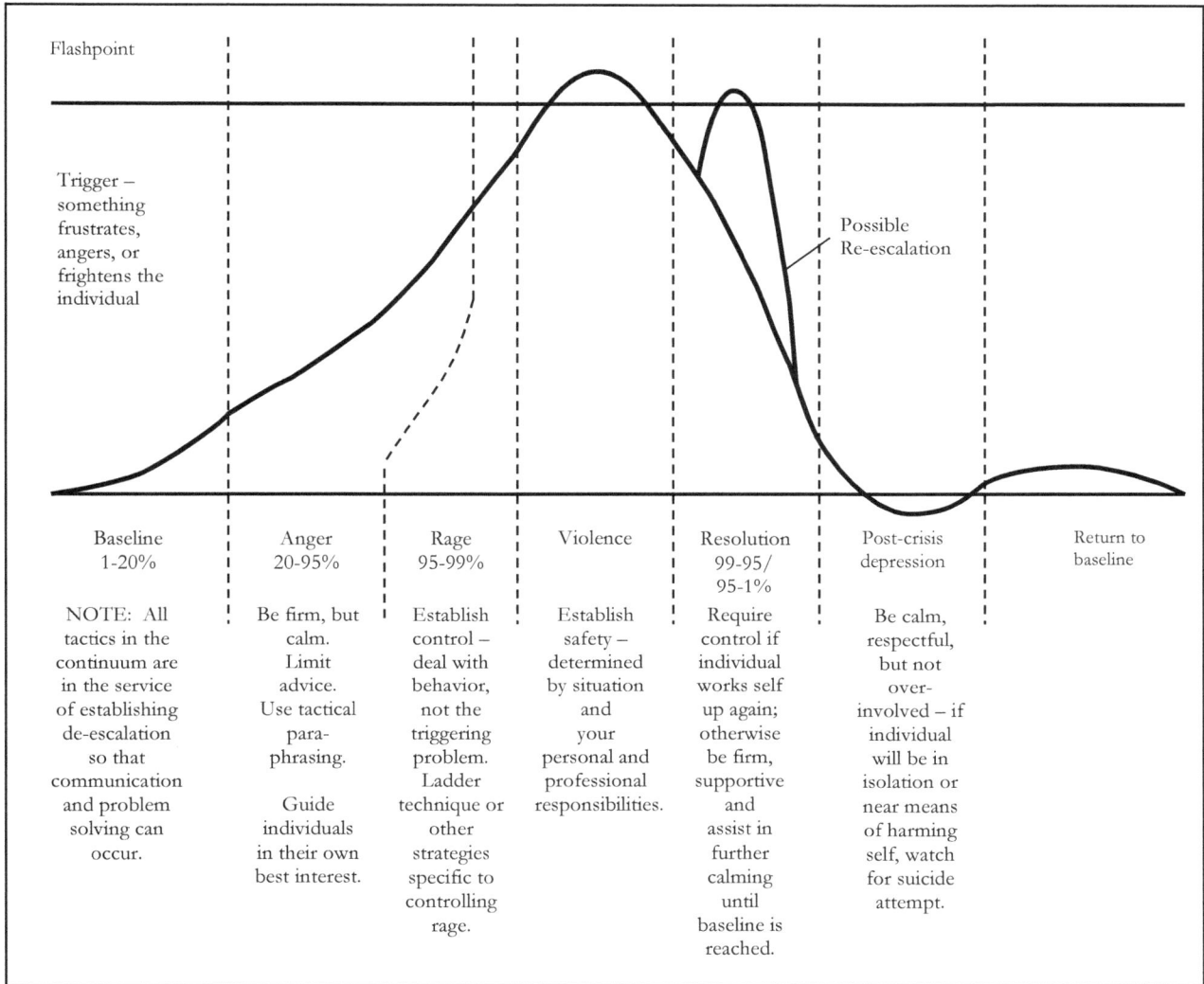

Flashpoint

Trigger – something frustrates, angers, or frightens the individual

Possible Re-escalation

Baseline 1-20%	Anger 20-95%	Rage 95-99%	Violence	Resolution 99-95/ 95-1%	Post-crisis depression	Return to baseline
NOTE: All tactics in the continuum are in the service of establishing de-escalation so that communication and problem solving can occur.	Be firm, but calm. Limit advice. Use tactical para-phrasing. Guide individuals in their own best interest.	Establish control – deal with behavior, not the triggering problem. Ladder technique or other strategies specific to controlling rage.	Establish safety – determined by situation and your personal and professional responsibilities.	Require control if individual works self up again; otherwise be firm, supportive and assist in further calming until baseline is reached.	Be calm, respectful, but not over-involved – if individual will be in isolation or near means of harming self, watch for suicide attempt.	

An outburst of aggression occurs in a cycle that starts with relative calm and ends with relative calm. Although the aggressive cycle often appears to start with a clear *triggering event*, the crisis may have been burning for some time beneath the surface. The reader may notice the term 'trigger,' being familiar with it in terms of substance-abuse relapse. In fact, they're similar. Many addicts have triggers that elicit the urge to use drugs; similarly, aggressive individuals, particularly the habitually violent, have triggers that cue them to become violent.

Calm/Baseline

When we're calm, we're at **baseline.** We use the parts of the brain most responsible for our better human characteristics: thinking, creativity, and forming social relationships. You can certainly have a fair amount of energy in a dialogue, and still be fully rational: a heated discussion, for example. For this reason, on a scale of 1 to 100, we approximate baseline as 1-20.

Anger

A triggering event elicits a change in both thinking and feeling. This event can be something that threatens a individual's sense of safety, infuriates him/her because they haven't gotten what they want, or are simply a cue that they're now justified using a skill (aggression) with which he/she is confident will allow them to achieve dominance or total victory. Once aggression is triggered, the person becomes irritable, then angry.

If violence is given the number "100" and baseline starts at "1" then ANGER is 20 through 95, with irritation at the low end of the scale. If the person at baseline is eminently human, the angry patient is a 'mammal.' The primary social focus for mammals is their place in a pack. It's the same for us human animals when we are frustrated, threatened, or believe we are being ill-treated. That is why angry people use such expressions as "I'm taking a stand," or "I won't be pushed around," or "Who do you think you're to talk to me that way!"

Nonetheless, the angry person is trying to communicate with us, although it is largely one-way. They may not care what we have to say, but they care very much that we get what *they* have to say. Because we perceive them to be obnoxious, domineering, or just plain irrational, we often discount what they're doing as communication. They, on the other hand, experience an increasing sense of frustration or desperation, and not infrequently, a sense of helplessness. From their perspective:

- When you don't agree with them, you're resisting what is clearly true or right. Certain patients cannot accept anyone disagreeing with them, experiencing it as a kind of attack.
- When you don't seem to grasp what they're saying, you're showing that you're disinterested, or too stupid to understand.
- When you don't comprehend what they are saying, you are implicitly accusing them of stupidity, because if they were 'smart enough,' you'd understand.
- When you don't agree or comply with them, you're frustrating them in achieving something they want.
- They have a sense of being wronged, experiencing a direct threat to their 'position,' as in, "You think you are too good to pay attention to me." Dominance hierarchy, for humans, includes not only one's position vis-à-vis others, but also one's self-image.

As people become more agitated, the areas of their brain that mediate basic emotions take over. At this point, equity, negotiation, or compromise becomes less and less attractive. In their frustration, patients shift to attempting to dominate you—to *make* you see things their way, or to comply with them. Their domineering behaviors are, as much as anything else, an attempt to 'get through' to you.

Think of arguments you have had when, frustrated, you said such things as: "No, that's not what I'm saying! Do I have to explain it again?" Or "Let me put it another way!" Or "You just don't get it! What do I have to say to make you understand?" Although counter-productive, you probably became more intense because you wanted the other person to grasp what you were saying.

Anger is accompanied by physical arousal, which functions as a feedback loop to drive the brain toward further arousal. When the heart rate rises 10 percent to 15 percent above baseline due to emotional excitement, angry people no longer care about the truth. We only care about being 'right' and proving others 'wrong.' Communication is seen as a 'win-lose' situation. We interrupt more frequently and cut other people off; we only listen to others to pick out the flaws in their argument.

Tactical communication with an angry person, particularly one who is mentally ill, focuses on '<u>LINING UP</u>' with them, tactics usually referred to as de-escalation strategies. <u>You prove that you comprehend what they're trying to say</u>. In other words, you're taking them seriously. This in itself is powerfully disarming, not only calming them down, but also helping you to work together to actually solve the problem.

Rage

Rage is a set of behaviors, including both physical actions and verbalizations that serve to disinhibit people so that nothing holds them back from violence. They are no longer trying to communicate—they're working themselves up to an attack. Their rage is almost instinctive; they desire to destroy, not merely become dominant. Some people slowly build themselves into a state of rage; others lash out violently with seemingly no prior warning, verbal or otherwise. Usually, however, even non-communicative aggressors will signal their rage through their body language and other non-verbal forms of communication. Firefighters and EMTs should be aware of these warning signs of impending assault, as manifested on the intuitive level (Chapter 3) and based on observable behaviors, as described in the remaining sections of this book.

Human beings have various inhibitors that check the desire to commit mayhem upon another person. The prime inhibitors are:

- **A fear of consequences**. The fear of counterattack, legal consequences, social disapproval, and a host of other possible negative outcomes.
- **Morality**. Toxic ideologies, and cultures in general often define one or another type of person as less than human, and therefore 'fair game' for violence. Nonetheless, almost all human beings possess a core set of more principles, and when face with the vulnerability of another human being, face a 'demand' to treat them without violence.[26]
- **Self-image**. A man may see himself as the kind of person who doesn't hit women, make a public display of aggression, or lose control of himself.
- **The relationship**. A feeling of responsibility toward the other person—friendship, love, or family—may hold them back from violence. Many people (not all, unfortunately) see firefighters and EMTs as people whom one shouldn't assault.

- **Learned helplessness**. Some people, abuse survivors, for example, have tried to defend themselves in the past and have failed repeatedly. They may believe that they can't fight back. Their rage, however, is there. We have unlovely phrases like 'a cornered rat,' or 'the worm turns,' that describe a person who has suppressed their rage, sometimes for years, because fighting back always meant they would get hurt. Given enough frustration or threat, such people may explode in a fit of uncontrolled anger and violence.

In short, rage is a transitional phase between anger and violence. For this reason, we assign it the numerical value of 95-99. What is the difference between rage and violence? Anger is a rocket ship all fueled up with some fumes coming out, and the countdown initiated. Rage is right before lift-off. The rocket has not yet moved, but there are flames and steam billowing out, making a terrible roar, so loud the ground shakes. It is a roiling moment of explosive, tenuous equilibrium. Fuel could still be cut to the rocket engines so that it sits silent on the launching pad, but there are only a few moments to act, because the rocket is about to lift off.

What you should experience in the face of rage is fear. This isn't a bad thing. Fear tells us that we're in danger and that we must do something—NOW! Fear switches us on so that our emergency response systems are activated.[27]

Fear doesn't mean we won't be able to handle the aggressor. All fear really demands is attention. A sense of powerlessness, on the other hand, is a *conclusion* that some people believe when they experience fear. Imagine two people about to get punched. One feels a sense of helplessness, a crumbling inward. The other feels a sense of outrage and at that instant knows that they will somehow win. That person has an internal sense that even if the body is wounded, their spirit will never be overcome. Fear can and should be a call to arms, not a sign of defeat.

The proper response to rage (when retreat is not an option) is to establish <u>CONTROL.</u> This is not oppression—rather you are the eye in the center of the hurricane. You impose order by establishing authority and taking control.

Figure 38.1 The Difference Between Anger and Rage

Imagine someone hands you a huge plastic container. Through its translucent sides, you can see a dark, hairy shape, a Goliath Bird-Eater, the world's biggest spider. It rustles around the container, shifting in your hands like it's filled with mercury. Is it creepy? Sure it is. Is there any reason to be afraid? Not really. As long as the lid is on the container firmly, you are absolutely safe. This is the equivalent of anger. Internally you say, "I'd better keep the lid on this thing."

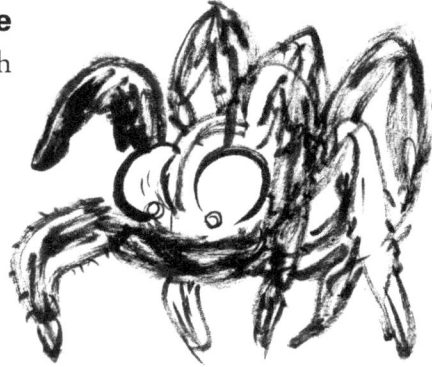

Now, imagine your 'friend' takes the container back, and to your surprise and horror, takes off the lid. The spider emerges onto the floor right next to your leg. It raises its front legs in threat-display and opens and closes its ¾ inch fangs. There is something poisonous, hairy, and mean in the room, and it is not enclosed in any container! The spider is out of the box. This, metaphorically, is rage.

However, the fear that now arises within you doesn't mean that you are helpless. You can step on the spider or jump up on a table. If you are ticked off enough, you can grab your 'friend' by the neck and make him sit on it! A belief that you are helplessness near the spider is an interpretation, not a fact. Fear is simply the warning cry—the drums at the brink of battle—that demands that you *must* act right now.

To deal with the enraged person, you must establish *control, especially if,* their behavior presents an immediate threat to you, to themselves, or to others. Control tactics—be they verbal or physical—are geared to establish the conditions that make the aggressive person no longer dangerous. In essence, using our metaphor above, we say, "Put the spider back in the box. Now!"

NOTE: There are, of course, many situations that the easiest solution is to escape. Verbal control tactics are used when that is not an options.

Violence

Violence doesn't begin when someone is hit or injured. Violence starts when you have good reason to believe that you or someone else is about to be hurt. It is violence when a patient has violated the 'safety zone' (the space between you at which you could credibly avoid an attack) and refuses to retreat. If the person doesn't have a weapon, we're talking about someone who is at about three arm's length distance and approaching in a menacing way. If armed, the distance can be much greater. Your guiding principle is <u>SAFETY,</u> which is defined by what you must protect. This includes yourself and other people for whom you're responsible.

This is when all your training comes into play. All your tools, be they verbal or physical, are at your disposal. There are definitely times when the firefighters and EMTs rightly decides that the best thing to do is to remove themselves from immediate threat, and return with back-up and the tactical advantage. Sometimes you hide and sometimes you act in an outlandish way that confuses the attacker. There are other times, rare though they may be, that the firefighter or EMT must use less-lethal or lethal force to be safe. You do whatever is most effective to protect yourself and the people around you.

CHAPTER 38

Why Would Someone
Become Aggressive?

Aggression is not an alien or unnatural emotion. Without a capacity for aggression, humanity would never have survived. Yet, much aggression seems far apart from the basic activities of hunting or self-defense. Why would someone be swept by rage when it causes so much harm? Why would people be prepared to throw away a future, even a life, driven by emotions that they themselves might be horrified to have expressed even a few moments later?

As you know from your own experience, there are many reasons to become angry or even enraged. We can better control aggressive people when we can communicate with them and we can do that better when we understand what set them off in the first place. Anger and rage can develop because a person:

- **Feels confused or disorganized**. They can't understand what is going on around them or 'inside' them due to cognitive distortions or a chaotic situation (too much information for them to figure out or put in 'order'). Among those who experience this confusion are those who are seriously mentally ill, autistic, developmentally disabled, intoxicated, or others who are overwhelmed by emotion, or an incomprehensible situation in which they find themselves. Imagine a huge net dropping onto you. You thrash and struggle chaotically trying to get free.
- **Feels helpless, enclosed, trapped, or overwhelmed**. This is similar in effect to disorganization, but it is accompanied by a particular anguish, because the patient usually perceives someone as the agent of their situation. This sense of desperation could be elicited by being stopped from leaving a situation, either physically or through psychological intimidation. For others, it is becoming enmeshed in an argument that gets worse and worse and continues to escalate. In the latter case, called 'emotional flooding,' people feel unable to speak sensibly and make others understand their point of view. This is most typically evoked in arguments between intimates where whatever one person says is 'checkmated' by the responses of the other.
- **Perceives an invasion of personal space.** Every human being has a sense of personal space (Chapter 7). If someone moves inside this space, the other patient will experience it as an attack. In volatile situations, no matter what your intentions, you will be perceived as an attacker if you step in another's personal space.
- **Demands what they perceive as justice.** It is rare that an angry person doesn't believe himself/ herself to be justified. Demands for justice are usually a complex sense of victimization or grievance and can include:
  a. *The patient feels that they're losing their autonomy and power.* In this case, the person feels dominated and oppressed, and regards themselves as fighting for their freedom. This sense of

loss of power is a personal reaction. It doesn't have to be 'true' in an objective sense, although not infrequently, a person's freedom is limited while an emergency is in process.

b. *The person feels that their rights are either denied, or being taken away.* Many people, mentally ill or not, experience a sense of violation when they're being limited or forced to conform to rules. Such patients believe that something that is vitally their own is being stolen away even when, in truth, it is for their own good.

c. *A 'self-appointed' revolutionary feels the world is unfair and rebels.* The best sense of power that many people can achieve is in opposition to others. In this sense, they welcome an opportunity to designate others as enemies: legitimate targets for their own hate. Paranoid people view themselves and others as being oppressed by systems or powers beyond them. They 'designate' you as a representative of those larger forces.

- **Becomes intoxicated.** A 'self-induced' delirium, intoxication causes poor judgment. For other people, drugs and alcohol aren't a 'problem'—they're a solution. They drink or take drugs to 'liberate' their brutal desires, something observed frequently among perpetrators of domestic violence.

- **Perceives a material threat.** People will fight to defend what they have or that to which they believe they're entitled. Many people regard violence as a legitimate response to the loss of one's home, job, or freedom.

- **Experiences organic stressors such as loss of sleep, insufficient or un-nutritious food, and/or fatigue.** Brain chemistry changes when the human organism is stressed. In turn, this causes changes in perception, mood, and cognition, and among these changes can be an increase in irritability or hypersensitivity.

- **Experiences emotional stressors and losses.** Anything that elicits profound emotion can cause a person to become volatile. This can include a recent loss through the death of someone close: job loss, divorce, infidelity, or feelings of profound insecurity. <u>Anything that would drive a person towards suicide can drive them towards violence as well.</u>

- **Feels a sense of entitlement.** For many people, entitlement is intertwined with desire. Their motto is, "If I want something, I deserve it, and if I'm not getting it, I have a right to be more forceful in my demands, so that it is given to me."

- **Responds to their ideology.** Religious and cultural factors, be they the larger culture of a society, religion, and nationality, or the smaller culture of a community or family, can provide an ideology that legitimizes aggression, even violence. Many cultures offer its members an 'operating system' that expects a violent response in certain situations. Furthermore, cultures often define certain people or classes as inferior, even less than human. All too many cultures sanction violence against women as a matter of course.

- **Is flamed up due to family interactions.** One of the biggest motivators of aggression is what occurs in families. There is the friction of arguments regarding everything from house rules to who 'owns' the house, irritation due to living too close together, past grievances brought up with no resolution, and a host of other issues. An argument starts, but it degenerates quickly into a demand that each concede that the other is right. Each feels flooded emotionally and becomes more and more irrational and furious because of their inability to 'get through' to the other. This becomes all the worse when one or more family member is mentally ill, because what they're arguing about may be irrational or delusional. Families often function as emotional traps: there is no escape from the people who, although loved, cause one the most pain.

- **Is flamed up due to things occurring within their romantic relationship.** People in relationships often demand that the other person submit to their wishes. There are numerous grounds to fight—money, sex, child care, infidelity, etc.

- **Has 'given up.'** For some, aggression, like its mirror-twin, suicide, is a 'problem-solving' activity or a 'what the hell' response when one can't find any other solution. Related to this is a person's belief that he/she has no effect on the world. Violence ensures that you will make an impact. Depressed people, particularly males, often manifest this type of aggression.

- **Hallucinates (command hallucinations).** The person is tormented by alien voices that assert an all-powerful identity. The person may feel compelled to comply with voices that urge violence, or in trying to make the hallucinations stop by any means, becomes violent. On other occasions, the voices, visions, smells, or sensations are simply distracting and irritating. Imagine a mosquito whining in each ear, crawling deeper into the ear canal: unreachable, unstoppable.

- **Feels shamed or humiliated.** One of the most powerful driving forces of aggression is a sense that one has been shamed. Shame isn't a mild sense of social embarrassment. It is a sense of being exposed and victimized by others, with no way to make it stop. It is a driving force for revenge-based aggression, and is also a prime motivator for attacks when a person identifies you with someone who shamed or violated them in the past. They may have been brooding about it for years, exploding into rage like an underground coal fire exposed suddenly to the air.

- **Has been set up by others.** This can occur for a variety of reasons:
  a. Family members or friends may provoke the aggressor. For example, a wife says, "I thought you were more of a man. You have to call an ambulance because of your chest hurting a little? You are such a baby!"
  b. Other people do this to *themselves* by 'fronting,' making a scene in front of others (friends or family, for example) to increase their status in their 'pack.' Out in front, they're afraid to back down. Others carry the 'audience' inside their imagination, demanding they conform to a 'macho' self-image.

- **Thinks "life is war."** Some criminals see themselves in a war, seeing anyone in uniform as a combatant on the other side of the lines, even the 'medics.'

- **Uses violence as recreation.** For some person, hurting others is perhaps the most pleasurable activity in their lives. There is a joy in making others submit, and for some, a delight in causing pain.

- **Uses surgical violence.** This is a conscious tactic of intimidation. "I won't hurt you if you do 'x' but if you don't do what I say, I will hurt you very badly."

- **Is acting out of protective rage.** This is the rage expressed by one trying to protect another perceived as being victimized. The closer one feels to the perceived victim, the more one's identity is 'merged' with them, and the more fiercely aggressive the 'protector' will be; for example, this can easily occur when a parent is nearby while you must do something frightening or painful to their child.

CHAPTER 39

What Does Escalation Look Like?

What do people do when they become aggressive? As people escalate, their bodies become activated to fight, to posture, to intimidate, or to flee. They can show a variety of different behaviors.

Mood Changes

- **Atypically withdrawn.** Some people avoid eye contact, stop speaking, or only respond with short phrases, or even monosyllables. This would only be relevant with a patient whom you see on a regular basis, who is showing a marked change in behavior from a more friendly norm. You should always 'assess' such patients, as in the following manner: "Arnie, this is the fourth time I've seen you this week. I know things hurt, but you always have a joke for me. This time when I greeted you, you turned your back, and now you are talking under your breath. Something's going on." Notice that you do not 'quiz' or question the patient; rather, you tell them what you observe and wait for a response. Angry people often interpret questions as either interrogation, or that you are so clueless that you don't see the obvious.
- **Nervous, anxious, even frightened.** Such people usually lash out in defense. They're not looking for a fight—they're trying to protect themselves.
- **Overwhelmed or disorganized.** Such a person begins to speak in repetitive loops or pace and babble or talk to themselves. This is a manifestation of intoxication or a chaotic mental state.
- **Hostile.** Hostility is the open expression of dislike, hatred or threat.
- **Seductive.** Seduction is when a patient tries to get you to collude with them, for example, "C'mon that's not abuse. You spank your kid when he gets out of line, don't you? You aren't going to call the cops on a spanking, are you?" Often this is just manipulation, but some people shift to overt violence when their 'masked aggression' fails.
- **Exhibits mood swings.** (Chapter 17) This means rapid shifts in mood, for example, boisterous and loud to morose, then shifting to depressed and quiet, to once again, loud, this time belligerent. Such patients present a particular risk, because they're both unpredictable and unable to control their own emotions.
- **Hypersensitive to correction or disagreement**. (Chapter 19) Hypersensitive people are very reactive to other people around them. They feel under perpetual attack. When there is no enemy, they will find one, or even create one. Paradoxically, they don't feel right with themselves unless they discover who is attacking them—in their world, someone always is.
- **React to authority issues.** These patients become very frustrated or outraged, refusing to comply with rules. Their motto of life can be summed up in the phrase, "No one can tell me what to do."

- **Electric tension.** This is that intuitive sense you get when you're approaching a dangerous situation, the feeling you get before a thunderstorm hits. (Chapter 7). **If you feel it, ALWAYS trust it,**

Changes in Thinking

- **Cognitive distortions.** Negative self-talk that makes the situation seem worse. Such cognitive distortions heighten the patient's belief that they're being abused or threatened.
- **Interpersonal cognitive distortions.** The person hears the worst possible interpretation in what another is saying. For example: "Tia, we're just going to call your psychiatrist to check on your medications." And her response is, "You're getting me committed again!!!!!!!"
- **Becoming less and less willing to negotiate.** The patient focuses increasingly on dominating the other, on winning the argument, or taking out their frustrations on the object of their anger rather than trying to find a way to a peaceful resolution.
- **Concentration and memory deteriorate.** It becomes more difficult for them to communicate, to solve problems, or to recall past problem-solving skills.
- **The angrier they are, the lower their ability to listen.** One focuses on being 'right,' not on finding out the truth. Without the ability to hear the other's perspective, they become either irrational or self-centered. In the latter case, only their own ideas and desires have any importance to them.
- **Judgment becomes worse and worse.** As their information processing skills deteriorate, their **judgment consequently becomes worse and worse.** They can't evaluate what is really in their own self-interest.

Figure 39.1 Example of impaired judgment due to escalated anger

One of the authors witnessed a man, angered at his wife, rip his IV needle out of his arm, tearing a laceration in the vein and spraying blood all over the emergency room.

Words or Lack of Words

- Behaving with morose, sullen **silence,** accompanied by hunched shoulders, knitted brows, and glaring at the floor or at other people.
- Becoming **sarcastic.** Sarcasm is hostility shaded in humor or passive-aggressive phrases. They jeer at you, or sneer scornfully, demeaning your strong attributes and highlighting your weak points.
- Becoming deliberately **provocative**, by doing and saying things to upset or irritate you. Provocation is a challenge, trying to elicit a response on your part that will justify them becoming increasingly hostile, if not violent. They twist what you say deliberately, trying to confuse you or make you feel ridiculous.
- Becoming increasingly **illogical**. This isn't like deliberate tactic of playing word games. Swept by anger, they misunderstand or misinterpret what you're doing or saying or veer off on a tangent whenever you try to offer calming words or a way to restore peace. They become unable to explain what they're doing or trying to say.

- Becoming **loud and demanding**, with a belligerent tone.
- Using **abusive or obscene language**.
    a. When the patient uses terms that are vile and degrading, they're trying to make you 'less than human.' They might not do violence to a human being, but because you're a _____ (fill in the blank), then it is no more wrong to be violent than it would to exterminate vermin or a wild beast.
    b. In other cases, the obscenities and slurs are a focused weapon. The aggressor uses the words to shock or stun, so that you focus on what they say and not on what they're simultaneously doing. While you're preoccupied with their vile language, you don't notice that they have shifted their feet and slipped a hand into their pocket.
    c. Note, however, that most people use obscenity as adjectives and punctuation. They swear to illustrate their own emotions and ideas, and truly aren't using their words as a form of attack. In the first two cases, you must deal with the verbal attacks as part of their mode of assault. In the latter event, correcting someone's rude way of speaking can escalate something that wasn't a problem in the first place.
- Making repeated **demands or complaints.** Of such people, we often say, "They have an attitude." This person is trying to legitimize a pervasive sense of grievance, so they have an excuse to argue or fight.
- **Refusing to comply** with rules or directives. In their mind, it is all or nothing. If they comply, they lose. Only resistance is victory.
- **Denying totally** either the facts or the implications of what they're doing. They're so angry that reality is irrelevant to them. They're right and you're wrong.
- Using **clipped, pressured speech**, thereby presenting as 'over-controlled,' even though they have the pent up energy of a volcano. Such people often use very formal or stilted language. "What do you mean, angry? What makes you think I'm angry. I am not angry. I will let you know when I'm really angry."
- **Implicit threats**. Boasts of past acts of violence or warns that they might not be able to stop themselves from doing what they did before.

Physical Organization—Disorganization

Facial Expressions. Facial expressions can vary a lot, depending on the mode of aggression. Facial expressions will be discussed in more detail in Section IX. The following list isn't hard-and-fast, but there is real likelihood when the following facial expressions are displayed the person means what follows:

- **Clenched teeth.** An attempt to contain or control intense emotions.
- **Bared teeth.** A threat display. You may have noticed some people smile who are really baring their teeth.
- **Grinding teeth.** A self-stimulating behavior used to internally escalate oneself.
- **Frowning.** Is often associated with anger, usually accompanied by a wrinkled forehead, and the eyebrows 'pulled together.'
- **Knitted brows.** The eyebrows are pulled together, and the person looks out from under the eyebrows, associated with smoldering anger.

- **Staring eyes.** (Particularly if there is tension in the cheeks and all around the eyes). Can be an attempt at intimidation or manipulation; targeting the other as prey.
- **Biting or compressing the lips.** Is associated with barely controllable intense emotions.
- **Quivering lips.** Is associated with fear or unhappiness.
- **Tightening the lips.** Is associated with an attempt to control or contain intense emotion.
- **Pulsating veins in the neck.** Is associated with building anger and rage.
- **Dilated pupils.** Is associated with drug intoxication.
- **Avoiding all eye contact.** When coupled with other expressions of aggression, this can be associated with planning an attack, hiding intentions of an attack, or, paradoxically, an attempt to disengage so that they won't be forced to fight.

Voiding. When angered, some people have an urge to void themselves, clearing their bodies for the fight. Nausea and vomiting can occur with reduced blood flow to the gut. Other people feel a need to urinate or an onset of diarrhea. These behaviors occur when a patient is in a state of intense fear or otherwise full of adrenalin.

Breathing.
- Those shifting into **offensive anger** often breathe deep in the chest and down into the belly. This can be slow or fast, depending on how fast their anger is building.
- Those going into **defensive aggression** usually breathe in a shallow, rapid, and irregular pattern—almost like panting or gasping. Some hyperventilate, breathing so fast that they go into an acute anxiety state. They may become violent out of a terror-induced panic.
- Sociopathic patients and others who are **'professionals' at violence** often maintain a smooth easy breathing pattern throughout.

Actions
- **Tense.** Most aggressive patients become tense and/or agitated. Sometimes people try to discharge the tension by pacing, usually typified by rapid jerky movements, or even exercise that clearly isn't for fun.
- **Posturing.** Those who are getting angry, as opposed to enraged, begin to posture, inflating the chest, leaning into the other, thrusting their chin forward. This is an intimidation pose rather than a fighting pose.
- **Fighting pose.** Some will take a fighting pose—a combative stance, as opposed to posturing, is often a crouch, with the chin tucked in. In other cases, the aggressor brandishes a fist or a weapon.
- **Relaxed.** One subset of aggressors, the predatory (Chapter 52), tends to relax when they're preparing for an attack. They're at home with violence, like a tiger or a snake. These people sometimes smile while making eye contact with you.
- **Implicit physical threats.** Hard eye contact, intrusion into your personal space, cracking knuckles, clenching fists, etc.

- **Ritualized behavior.** Men, in particular, though not exclusively, will begin to ritualize their behavior, going into a stereotypical 'war dance,' puffing up their chests and spreading their arms to make their torso look bigger, invading their 'victim's' personal space, pacing, smacking their fist in their hand, breathing faster, etc. They may move in quick jerky starts and stops, making movements toward their victim and then back, as if working themselves up to attack.
- **Positioning.** Those looking for a *fight or confrontation* square off directly in front of their target, while those looking for a *victim* tend to move on the target's corner, so that they can attack where they're vulnerable.
- **Glaring.** Some aggressors glare into your eyes with a direct hard stare
- **Trespassing.** Some aggressive patients will trespass on personal space, even 'accidentally-on-purpose' bumping into or jostling their prospective victim.
- **Power testing.** Picking up, mishandling, or even breaking the other's possessions. An example would be putting his feet on your vehicle.
- **Visual rape.** Some men use their eyes to trespass on women, running their gaze over their bodies in what is a 'visual rape.' The implicit communication is, "What I'm doing with my eyes, I could do with my body any time I wanted."
- **Displacement activity.** Hitting, kicking, or throwing objects. This is done to discharge tension, as a threat display and as a 'warm up.'
- **Scapegoating.** This is a form of displacement activity expressed on living beings rather than objects. For example, a man, furious with an EMT, screams at his wife, "Would you shut that damn kid up!"
- **Making a dramatic scene.** The patient 'acts crazy,' either to get closer to you than you'd let someone who was purposefully targeting you, or to get you so preoccupied with calming them down so you lose sight of larger tactical concerns.

The Edge of Attack

- Angry or otherwise emotionally upset people have a flushed face: the pale-skinned turn red, and the dark-skinned turn even darker. In essence, blood at the surface of the skin is threat display, as if to say, "See how ANGRY I am!" If people blanch—light-skinned people turn bone-white, and dark-skinned people get a grayish tone—this indicates RAGE. The threat is not potential: it is <u>now</u>. Note, however, that many intoxicants flush the face, so that this is not a reliable metric to assure you that the patient is 'merely' angry.
- Increased **pacing**, while muttering to oneself, is arousing, bringing oneself closer and closer to the edge or attack
- Some people engage in **more and more displacement activity**, hitting, kicking, and throwing things.
- Others will **internalize** all signs of incipient assault, and thus, it seems to come out of nowhere. Right before the attack, these people momentarily stop breathing. They can be utterly quiet and still—the 'calm before the storm.' It's as if you aren't there. In the latter case, the patient will sometimes have a 'thousand-yard stare,' where they seem to look beyond or through you.

- Some people, particularly, but not exclusively, the psychotic aggressor, get an **eerie smile** on their face, one that holds no mirth.
- As the attack is incipient, the aggressor can **'lose it'**—shaking, yelling, and acting berserk.

Explosion and Resolution

The crisis will be some form of assault, either verbal or physical. Of course, at this point, you will do whatever you must do to establish safety. After the explosive episode, the aggressor moves to the **resolution** phase in which they gradually, sometimes very gradually, returns to baseline. Their body relaxes, cognitions improve, and their actions are less stereotypical. After resolution, there is often a **post-crisis depression**, which is due partly to physical depletion (the stored nutrients in the body are used up), and is partly psychological. The patient may be remorseful, apologetic, resentful, or merely withdrawn (Chapter 55).

SECTION VIII

De-escalation of
Angry Patients

CHAPTER 40

Core Principles Of Intervention
With Angry People

Figure 40 Techniques for angry patients

All the techniques in this section are for angry patients (mentally ill or not). Some work for low to moderate anger (irritation), and others across the entire range of anger. Remember they are a response to the angry person's attempts to communicate. We control them by establishing that we 'got' the communication, so that there is no longer any need for the anger.

Note that methods used to de-escalate angry people don't work with enraged people. In fact, they will very likely further escalate the situation. Imagine saying to the berserk methamphetamine intoxicated psychotic, "I see you want to rip my brains out of my skull and smear them on the walls. You've been having a rough day today."

Conversely, using strategies that are suitable for enraged people (control tactics) with angry people will flame them upwards *into* rage. Imagine coming home and your spouse tells you that he/she is not happy at all that you forgot the groceries in the trunk of the car, and you say, "Step back. Give me five feet right now!" (It's going to be a long night, isn't it?)

When dealing with potentially aggressive patients, safety must supersede all other concerns. If you don't establish safety for yourself and others, you can be of no assistance to anyone. This doesn't mean that you shouldn't be talking with the aggressive patient, reassuring them, or negotiating. However, everything you do must have a tactical basis: even reassurance or validation is in the service of safety. Solving problems must wait until safety is established. In the material that follow, there are page after page of techniques for de-escalation. Some are widely applicable, whereas others may only be useful in very specific situations. This is a catalog of techniques, not a sequential series of procedures. Think of them like the scales and octaves of music that must be mastered so that you can improvise freely.

- **Knowledge.** Obtain as much information as possible from dispatch. Be aware there are other individuals with scanners listening to your radio transmission including the media, so the dispatchers must be educated how best to convey information without compromising a patient's privacy. Attempt to use your cell phone to obtain protected patient information from the dispatcher; however, if there is a danger to all of the responding departments, radio transmission is acceptable to warn of any dangers known by the dispatch center.

- **De-escalate, then solve the problem.** Your focus should be on what the patient is doing, not the cause of the upset. <u>You can't solve a problem with an angry person</u>. De-escalate first and minimize the anger—then engage in problem solving.
- **Watchful waiting.** Sometimes the best control tactic is letting them control themselves. You remain centered and ready as the angry person calms himself/herself without any assistance from anyone else. This doesn't mean that you ignore them. You're ready to suppress any action on their part that would indicate that they're ramping up instead of down.
- **Trust your hunches.** If you have a vague sense that something is wrong, you're probably right. You're becoming aware of the first behaviors that they display when getting angry (Section II).
- **Only one person should talk to the angry patient.** Trying to talk to two or more people at once will cause the angry person to become more and more confused, as well as making him feel attacked and surrounded. <u>Your fellow responders need to learn to be patient with the patient.</u> If you are pacing the discussion to the patient's response, it is important the other first responders don't interrupt the interaction with extra questions. If any first responder violates this precept, it must be a subject in after-action review. If you have a problem with law enforcement officers contributing their input when a firefighter or EMT should have the lead in communication, this usually has to be addressed, supervisor to supervisor. It must be addressed, however, because everyone's safety is on the line.
- **Be what you want them to be.** Embody exactly how you want them to behave: calmly, with slow breathing, and upright posture. People tend to mirror the behavior of the most powerful patient with whom they're interacting. If you are out of control, the angry person will be even more so. Conversely, if you're calm and powerful, other people tend to calm as well.

CHAPTER 41

Physical Organization In the
Face Of Aggression

How you stand, how you breathe, how you use eye contact, your gestures, and your posture are all essential factors in calming aggressive people. You can say all the 'right' things, but if you look like you're afraid, irritated, or angry, your verbal interventions will have no effect whatsoever and the situation will only get worse.

Breathe with your entire torso, not high in your chest. When you breathe rapidly with your chest, you tend to hyperventilate, which 'informs' the brain that you're in trouble because *you need more oxygen now!* Deep, powerful chest breathing, on the other hand, excites the more primal areas of the brain: not flight, but fight. We strongly recommend that you master 'circular breathing,' (Chapter 8) to help you modulate and control internal agitation. However, for those who aren't able to effectively use circular breathing, or when one has to teach people in a short time, a more simple method is to inhale on a six count, pause your breath on a two count, and exhale on a six count, As described in the last chapter, people tend to calm around people who are powerfully calm themselves. Proper breathing is the quickest avenue towards that end.[28]

Be at an angle to the upset person. Standing, this is sometimes called a 'blade stance,' because you stand with one foot in front of the other, the back foot at a 30 - 45 degree angle with some space between them (don't put the two feet in one line!). Paradoxically, this is both calming (as people can tolerate your proximity better than if you were standing 'squarely,' confronting them), and also a much better stance to appear and feel strong (because you're both more balanced, and better prepared to protect yourself from a blow or a kick). If you have anything on your belt that might be used against you as a weapon, that side of your body should be 'bladed away' from the patient.

If you're seated. You can still use a 'blade stance while seated.' Sit on the edge of the chair, with the lead foot flat on the floor, and the other on the ball of the foot. You don't look ready to fight, but you are. You simply look relaxed and alert, and you can get to your feet without your hands, thereby being able to employ them in any way necessary.

Use the stillness of your hands as a calming agent. Clasp your <u>wrist</u> with the other hand. You can stand this way relaxed for a long time. By clasping your wrist, you slightly broaden yourself, and you will feel solid rather than nervous. Furthermore, you're ready to bring your hands upwards to fend off or block a strike *without looking like you're ready to do so*. In other words, there is no apparent fight in your stance, just strength. It is being tactical without looking tactical.

Use your hands as a calming fence. You can use your hands as a fence in a 'natural' way by 'talking' with them. The hands are held up in front of the chest, with the backs of the hands forward, one hand in the palm of the other. Keep what movements you make with your hand and arms slow and small. You're rotating your elbows, not swinging your arms from the shoulders. Agitated people will become more so if the firefighter or EMT is waving his/her arms in what appears to be threatening or chaotic gestures. If the situation is getting more heated, and the person is increasingly encroaching in your space, turn both of your hands, palms out, in front of you to set a boundary between you and the angry person. The arms should angle from the body at about 30 degrees, and the hands should be relaxed and curved slightly. *Both the hands and arms should be relaxed, like a flexible willow branch rather than like iron bars.* Of course, you can use these upraised hands to push back away or fend off if you have to. The hands shouldn't be in a 'fighting stance' nor stiff in a rejecting gesture.

Figure 41.1 Don't use only one hand unless the danger is high

When trying to de-escalate someone when the situation is not too heated, holding up *one* hand is more likely to provoke the patient. Rather than a fence, a single hand becomes the leading point of a triangle, your shoulders being the other two points. Many people experience this as aggression on your part. That one hand is 'in their face.'

Be aware and sensitive to body spacing.

- Don't get so wrapped up in communicating with them that you're unaware of their agitation. They may be shifting back and forth, looking down or away, begin to tremble, have their eyes go flat, or sway backwards. (Chapter 7).

- Are they too close to you? If they keep trespassing in your body space, tell them that you're happy to talk about the problem, but they should step back—they're standing too close. For example, if the person escalates and steps forward, turn your hands outward to accompany your verbal setting of a limit (For example, "Mr. Jackson, I want to hear what you are saying, but you are standing too close. Keep talking to me, but take a few steps back.")

- Try to distinguish between the mentally ill patient, who is unconsciously too close (and needs to be taught space issues), and the person who is consciously trespassing. Don't forget, mentally ill people can be aggressive or predatory as well!

- As escalation and danger increase, establish the ideal space to create an authoritative presence so as to keep yourself out of harm's way and most effectively control the other person. Not too close or too far away. This is generally two arm lengths apart with adults. With small children, try to assume a low posture, so that your head heights are equal.

Figure 41.2 One author's experience: intercultural rules of spacing

Various cultures have different 'rules' regarding physical proximity and distance. To make matters more complicated, people within any culture are more diverse than you could possibly imagine. For example, I lived in Japan for well over a decade. It is a truism that people from East Asia don't like direct eye contact as much as people from America. This was certainly accurate with most people. However, I have had some Japanese people stare so deeply in my eyes that I felt like they were counting the wrinkles in my brain. So don't assume that someone is close to you "because they're from 'x' culture." Someone *from* 'x' culture may be getting close to you with the intention of harming you, just like someone from your own.

To be sure, you should be aware of cultural conventions so that you don't unnecessarily offend people. At the same time, such patients are now living in this culture (wherever my reader resides) and therefore, in setting your own limits regarding space, you are teaching them how better to survive in their new home. Therefore, if someone is too close for your comfort, whatever culture they're from, tell them tactfully to move back so that you can continue your conversation with more ease, and conceivably, safety.

Try to breathe and move slowly and smoothly. Agitated people startle easily. If you're breathing slowly and moving smoothly, however, they will tend to calm in rhythm with *you.*

The art of eye contact. In almost all cases, it is best to have direct eye contact with the angry patient you're trying to calm. You must be both non-threatening and non-threatened. In other words, to use your eyes to calm someone else, you must show that calm and strength in your own eyes. You are NOT 'staring them down.' There are several exceptions to the eye-contact rule:

- Some psychotic or disorganized people find eye contact to be very invasive. **When they're calm or only slightly agitated,** angle your body in such a way so that they don't feel confronted or forced to make eye contact with you. If they escalate into real aggression, however, you must make eye contact to establish control, whether they're mentally ill or not.

- There is a disinterested "no-eye-contact" that can be used with *aggressive-manipulative* people (Chapter 51).

- There are some people who are so frightening that you feel your will is breaking and your mind taken over when you make eye contact with them. Others are so chaotic, manipulative, or confusing that you find yourself unable to maintain a solid sense of what to do or say when you make eye contact. If you're facing either of these types of patients, look between their eyes at the skin of their forehead. When you look into someone's eyes, you're establishing a human connection. If that connection puts you off-balance, then it's dangerous to you. When you look at their forehead, you're just looking at layers of dead skin. You will find yourself far calmer, and the patient, *if aggressive,* will still think you're looking in their eyes. You will just appear very strong.

CHAPTER 42

Tone And Quality Of Your Voice
For De-escalation

Talk as a professional. An angry person will focus on your tone rather than the content of your words. Don't betray any negative or angry emotions. For example, a bored tone with either impatience or condescension is guaranteed to evoke more anger, not less.

In most situations, try to pitch your voice a little lower than is usual for you. Under stress or intimidation, our voices tend to go up in pitch. When you pitch your voice lower, you will feel a little vibration in your chest. You get immediate feedback that you have taken control of your own body. In addition, a quiet, but strong, low-pitched voice—only a little lower than normal, not necessarily a baritone—communicates that control to the aggressor. This is the voice you use to deliver strong unambiguous verbal commands.

Slow down. It is often useful to speak a *little* slower than they do. However, don't speak in slow motion or in such a way that they think you're trying to hypnotize them. You're trying simultaneously to get them to resonate with your slower energy and also to keep yourself from being swept up in theirs. (As will be described below, there are other times that you want to 'catch' the other person up in your energy. In these cases, you may speak with speed and/or enthusiasm.)

Don't be 'saccharine.' Unless you're dealing with a small child in distress or someone severely developmentally disabled, don't use a soft, nurturing voice. When you talk to people as if they're children, incapable, helpless, and/or fragile, they will either feel that way, or feel that you're trying to make them that way. People who feel incompetent believe that they can't make things better. This includes calming themselves down. That overly sweet vocal tone can provoke the aggressor to regress to a more child-like state, which can easily deteriorate into hysteria or a tantrum, which in an adult body means an assault. Others, insulted at what they perceive as condescension, become angrier.

When necessary use a dramatic voice. When should you use it? It will feel like the right thing to do. Make your voice a little louder, and use charisma to grab attention.

Figure 42.1 Example of the use of a dramatic voice

A mentally ill woman, with a child-like presentation, is upset because she thinks people in the apartment lobby are laughing at her. You say, "Claire, I SEE you are upset! I'D be upset too if I thought those people were laughing at me! Now COME ON over here!" Indicate with your body where you want her to go, moving as if you are absolutely certain she will comply. "C'mon. I want you to tell me EXACTLY what happened! EVERY word! Let's go over here where no one can bother us!"

Show her that not only are you giving her your complete attention, but the drama means that she is important, the center of the action. By moving her somewhere else to talk, you remove her from the scene that is upsetting her.

When to use the "battle cry." With few exceptions, the major time you would be yelling at a patient is combat. This is the battle cry, an emergency shout of "NO!" or "FREEZE!" or "STEP BACK!" You only use this when an aggressor is attacking you or otherwise presenting immediate danger to someone. You roar like a lion to startle and momentarily freeze their motion, so you can evade attack and escape, put them in custody, or deploy a weapon on them while they aren't moving.

- Open your eyes WIDE!
- Slam your stomach BACK to try and connect your navel and your spinal column.
- Tighten your throat. (This will be a little painful to some people, leaving a raw throat for the next day, but it's worth it if it saves you or someone else from harm).
- **ROAR** a command.

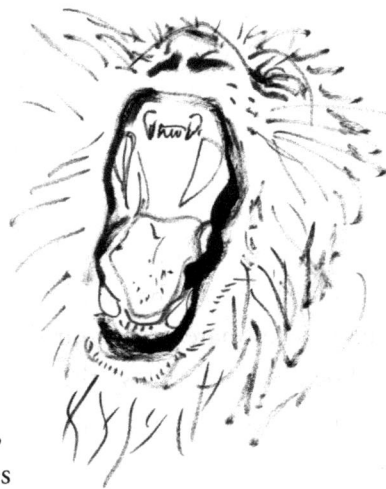

Figure 42.2 The choice of words for a battle cry

When an attacker, already close to you, is moving toward you with hostile intent, don't command that they "Stop!" or "Freeze!" They may comply and still be too close. Instead, command that they **"Step Back!"** or **"Move Back!"** or **"Back Off!"**

The commands **"Stop!"** or **"Freeze!"** should be used to arrest an action that will, in itself, result in harm; for example, if an attacker is about to assault another person, throw something, or simply run out into traffic. You are trying to shock them into momentary immobility, so that you can effectively get hold of them or deploy a weapon to stop their threat.

CHAPTER 43

Dealing With People Across The Spectrum Of Anger

Sometimes an early intervention moves a patient to a state of calm. You avert the crisis before it happens. You will surely remember incidents when you interacted with angry people, mentally ill or not, where one or another of the interventions in this chapter fits the situation.

An attitude of calm. An essential factor to lining up with the aggressive patient is *your* attitude. They're in an emergency state and believe there is no time left. If you also believe there is no time, you're both in crisis and you won't be able to act as a stable person to help them get back to a peaceful state.

Greet them and work your way towards them. In a situation where a patient appears to be brooding or preoccupied about a grievance or perhaps a delusion or obsession, it is often not a good idea to immediately start talking about what you believe is upsetting them, or unless they are in a clearly emergent state, jumping right in to treat them. Instead, start with a greeting. Introduce yourself. Explain why you are there, and what you do. It's common courtesy. This is also an informal assessment tool: if they resist your attempt to redirect them, this informs you right away that the situation is potentially serious.

Use a "door opener." State in an impartial way what you observe or believe is disturbing them. For example, 1) "You looked like you are having a bad day." 2) "Something just happened between you and that cop. I saw you guys talking when we arrived." Notice that in both cases you don't ask if there is something wrong or a problem. When you ask a question, you give the person an opportunity to simply close the door by denying what you observe. An open-ended statement implies that it is self-evident, as if to say, "We're already past the argument whether my perception is real or not. At this point, we're discussing what this perception means to you and to me." Follow this question with *silence*, accompanied by an open inquiring expression on your face, as if the next move—their reply—is a given.

Don't make sudden moves, unless the fight has started. A sudden move may be interpreted as an attack. When you move with measured calm, you slow the process, and hence the patient down.

Tell me—you don't have to show me. As elementary a suggestion as this might sound, the following illustrates the power of this intervention. A very upset patient begins swearing at an EMT. She replies, "Al, it is absolutely clear that you're upset. Furious! And I'm able to help you with this. But I can't and won't do that when you swear at me. Tell me why you're upset. You don't need to show me."

Demonstrate empathy. Empathy isn't the same as sympathy, that feeling of sorrow for the person's plight. Empathy simply means that you grasp, approximately, what other people are feeling based on their physical organization, what they are saying and how they say it. Use phrases such as, "I understand you are…." or; "What you're saying really makes sense," or; "I imagine I'd feel the same way….". We thereby demonstrate that we grasp what the person is experiencing without necessarily agreeing with it.

Figure 43 Don't overdo empathy

There are some de-escalation systems that make this a centerpiece of their training methods. However, if you overuse this you will sound like a parody of a 'therapist in an asbestos coat.' Like everything else we have discussed, it is a tactical communication that is to be used sparingly at just the right time.

Let them tell their story. Sometimes people simply have to say their piece. There is no need to problem-solve and no need to interrupt. In such cases, listening with attention and respect is all that they need.

Be professional. Professional distance gives the patient a clear understanding of the true nature of your relationship with them.

Ask what kind of help they need. Of course, you can ask questions if a person is only mildly upset. Ask what they want or need. If you have a solution to the problem, explain it clearly to them, give them an idea how long it will take and what they should do in the interim. If you can't solve the problem, tell them who can, or what they must do next. Always try to explain the process. Many folks walk around frustrated. With the proper information they de-escalate on their own. This is particularly valid with service-level complaints.

Team up with them. Incorporate them into your 'team' by using the word 'we.; When they accept this unconsciously, they begin to feel that they're working with you, not against you. A couple of examples are: "Let's you and me sit over here." And, "Yes, we do have a problem. Let's see what we can do to figure this out."

Give. Some EMTs have a stuffed animal to give to smaller kids to hold while they are treating them (the kid gets to keep the stuffed animal!).

Humor. This is the ability to see a situation from another perspective, can sometimes work like magic. However, you must be very careful—it only is helpful when the person is at low levels of irritation rather than strong anger. If they're too upset or agitated, their response to a joke or humorous comment is likely to be, "You're making fun of me," or "This is serious. You think this is a joke?"

Distract. Particularly with young or cognitively impaired people, it is often best to simply distract them. This is sometimes useful even with people who are in a delirium state, where you distract them long enough so that they can safely be restrained. Their anger is driven by feelings and sensations, rather than by what they're thinking. If you can change the focus of their attention, their anger often dissipates.

Honesty is golden. Don't promise what you can't do or otherwise try to fool the person. If you suggest a solution to the problem, be clear what the limitations are. Many people take negotiation as concession, believing they will get everything they demand. If they don't clearly understand their options, they will later experience a sense of betrayal when they're refused something they want.

CHAPTER 44

Diamonds In The Rough—
Essential Strategies For
De-escalation Of Anger

Codes of Living

People live by codes, and paradoxically, those leading outlaw lifestyles cling to codes most of all. Some of those codes are based on the culture into which they're born, and others are based on the culture or lifestyle they adopt. Some of these codes are passed down within a family, while other people may create a code in resistance to the codes they were bequeathed. Some people's codes are impeccable principles of personal integrity, while others are eccentric rules congruent only with their mental illness or character disorder.

The heart of their code is often a phrase of one or two words that sums up their deepest values. When people talk about themselves, their codes of living are often woven throughout their speech. This is especially true when people are angry. The reason for their outrage is often their belief that their code is being threatened or compromised:

- They perceive that others are demanding they violate their code.
- They take offense when others don't conform to their code.
- They think another's actions require them to respond or they will violate their code.

Angry people will very often proclaim their code for living in a tirade.

Figure 44.1 Examples of patients proclaiming codes and values

Person 1. "I'm a man. He can't talk about me that way."

Person 2. "Think of how I feel. If someone did that to you, wouldn't you be upset?"

Person 3. "Are you saying I'm not going to get paid? I did the job and you owe me. Whether you like it or not isn't the issue, you owe me!"

Person 4. "I was standing there all alone. Everyone was looking at me. Talking about me!"

You should be able to describe their code in one or two words. What is most important to each of these people in the above examples? Patient #1 is focused on pride; #2 on empathy, that others should understand his situation; #3 is focused on obligation and an implicit contact being broken; and #4 is focused on humiliation.

This code is an access route to the person. When you incorporate it in your response, they feel understood. Another way to think of this is that you're filtering out the static and noise to get to the real music. Take note of the following:

- **Personal integrity.** Frame your suggestions with the same theme. "I wouldn't want people talking about you as a man who can't control himself."
- **Respect.** "Man, I can see how angry you are. I'd be angry too if someone said that to me. But if you assault him, you would be letting him 'own' you. He says three words, and you end up getting arrested, and maybe losing your job. No, I'm not saying to let it go. Let's you and me figure something out, so you win in a real way, and still keep your respect."
- **Situational.** The dominant metaphor here is that it is 'hot and tired.' "Look, Frank, I know it's a hot day, I'm tired, and I guess you are. I don't care who's right here, really; I just want to finish this paperwork so you can get the treatment you need from the hospital. These hot days are a killer. Here you and I are stressed out, just cause it's so miserable out here."
- **Tunnel vision.** A person can get so focused on an issue that it is all they can think about. "Disgusting. Absolutely right. Those meds are disgusting. They must taste terrible, and don't let anyone tell you different. If they didn't work so well, the doctor would never tell you to take such disgusting tasting things. But they do work, don't they?"

Break the Pattern

An aggressive person, set on conflict, often attempts to enmesh you in an inescapable system. Consider the following:

- **Aggressive man.** "What are you looking at?" "Nothing," replies the intimidated other person. "What!!!! You called me nothing!!!?'
- **Aggressive man.** "What are you looking at?" "I just looked in your direction," replies the intimidated other person. "What!!!! There's something on my face you don't like!!!? Or are you just calling me ugly?"

In 'breaking the pattern,' you do or say something that makes continuing the dispute absolutely impossible. In many cases, you will use a dramatic voice or display somewhat uncharacteristic or outlandish behaviors. It is hard to describe *how-to* do this. Let us show you, instead:

Figure 44.2 One author's experience of breaking the pattern

A man came into a clinic, drunk and belligerent. I came out and yelled, "Man, WHAT have you been DRINKING? Me – I like Ten Canes Rum. Whoa, <holding up two hands and yelling boisterously> Not your turn yet! I'm talking about my rum! Ten stalks of sugar cane for one bottle of rum. It is as golden as a tiger's eye and SWEET as sin. Man, I love my rum. I go home, take two ice cubes and put them in a glass. When the rum hits that ice, I hear a crack as clear as the bell in a church and I know everything is going to be alright, because I worship in the church of rum!"

What have YOU been drinking?"

He blearily looked at me and said, "White port."

"What KIND of white port. I need to know WHAT you have been drinking!"

"White port, I dunno." he slurred out.

"AHH man, not white port! Sit down here and tell me why you've been drinking that stuff."

We ended up sitting on two chairs, laughing and talking about our favorite drinks, until the police arrived and escorted him out.

Breaking the Pattern seems like magic, a highly developed intuitive skill that some of us imagine we would never be able to do. You can't have an array of special catch-phrases ready to disarm any aggressor. It is pure improvisation, like jazz or rap. The key isn't how creative you are, as if only brilliant people can possibly bring this off. It is actually the outcome of the same powerful calm that we have written about throughout this manual. When you're *trying* to be creative, you may say something witty, but it will be at the wrong time, with the wrong timing, and to the wrong person. When you're in control of yourself, with the mainline skills of de-escalation at hand, such improvisation will simply emerge, an idea or sentence that 'demands' to be said. You will be **wrong**, off-center, or off-target if you're *excited* about what a cool or funny thing you're about to say. Although the story you tell later about what you said may be dramatic or hilarious, you aren't a comedian trying to be entertaining. We can't teach you how to 'break the pattern'—however, if you've been reading this book, you'll have learned how to calm yourself, and thereby, how to put yourself in a mindset that you'll know how to do it yourself.

Figure 44.3 Example of the use of humor to break the pattern

A police officer was arresting a drunk when he called her that word that, more than any other, makes many women incensed. With a look of puzzlement on her face, she said, "Jimmy, do you spell that with a K or a C? I need it for my paperwork."

"K," he replied.

She answered, "Jimmy, if you are going to use big boy language, you should at least know how to spell it. It starts with a C."

He responded "It does? Damn, they didn't teach me that one in school."

Silence

Sometimes the most powerful thing you can do is to be silent. Be sure that you aren't being passive-aggressive, or fuming in silent anger. Instead, you're powerfully, quietly waiting. Such silence can evoke curiosity, anxiety, or a desire for a response. Keep your face calm, your posture centered, and be aware and truly interested. Calmly nod your head as you listen. Do this slowly and only several times—intermittently. In many cultures, including America, if you nod your head too rapidly and often, it means that you want the other person to hurry up and finish, or simply shut up.

Silence, however, isn't that easy. There are three ways to listen silently, and two of them will make people very angry.[29]

Contemptuous silence. You're tired of the dispute, or may be tired of the person. You fidget, you sigh, and most significantly, you twist one corner of your mouth, and roll your eyes upwards to one side. In all cultures that we're aware, this facial expression and behavior expresses the attitude that you hold the other in complete contempt. It is guaranteed to provoke rage.

- **Stonewall silence.** When you stonewall, you ignore the person or make it clear that you wish they would shut up. You can also appear to do this inadvertently when you're inputting data, listening on the phone simultaneously or to another conversation, or taking notes. Stonewalling evokes incredible anxiety in the other who wants to get through to you, finding that there's a 'wall' in the way. They will do anything to get "through," and this includes yelling, hitting, or begging.

- **Interested silence.** *The Right Way.* When you have been listening well, the angry person often ends up asking, "Aren't you going to say something?" or "Don't you have any ideas?" If they don't ask, and continue to talk and talk— interrupt them. Do this by advancing a hand slightly at your waist level or a little higher, fingers curved, palms down (you don't want the patient to interpret your hand movement as a 'shut up' gesture). Your shoulder also leans in just a little. In effect, almost subliminally, you're indicating that it's your 'turn.' In either event, you say, "I *do* have something to say." **The first thing you should do is to sum up your understanding of what he just said. You have to prove that you were listening.** This becomes the perfect lead-in to "tactical paraphrasing" (Chapter 45). If they're talking really intensely, put up both palms, open your eyes wide, and say something like, "Okay man, okay! It's my turn."

Some people find staying silent difficult, particularly when the other person is talking nonsense, or making a fool out of themselves. Remember this is a tactic: if nothing else, be interested as a 'street scholar,' studying how people can come up with the things that they're saying.

CHAPTER 45

Tactical Paraphrasing— The Gold Standard With Angry People

Paraphrasing is perhaps the most important technique for calming **angry** people. You sum up in a phrase or sentence <u>your understanding</u> of what the angry person has just said in a paragraph. If you paraphrase accurately, you have established that you have 'gotten' it that far, so they don't have to repeat it or try to say it in other words. It is like peeling off a single layer of an onion so that you can be shown the next one. If you don't show that you 'get' it, the angry patient will feel compelled to repeat and/ or elaborate that layer of the problem with more and more intensity. As they get more intense, they usually get more irrational, and their ability to communicate breaks down even further. The wonderful thing about paraphrasing is that you don't have to be 'smart' and interpret anything. You simply have to listen carefully.

Returning to our image of an onion, as you peel off each layer, they get to the next layer that is driving them. They might start out complaining about a pain in their hip, and that paraphrased—tell you that their wife left, and that paraphrased, start talking about suicide.

Paraphrasing establishes that you're truly listening and have understood what they have said. There is another component however where we also take a slightly activist approach. We *select* what we will paraphrase, choosing the healthiest aspect of what the angry person has just said.

This method is 'self-correcting,' whereas passive summation can make things worse.
- If you sum up an angry person's worst impulses, they may find themselves in full agreement with you, and escalate further.
- If you sum up an aspect of what they have said that is in the direction of conflict resolution, you will draw out of them that which *does* wish to resolve the conflict.
- On the other hand, if they're, in fact, bent on mayhem, they will correct you by escalating what they're saying, believing that you aren't getting the message.

Remember, they're trying to communicate! All you have to do is sum up what you understand from what they said. When you get it right, they go to the next layer.

Figure 45.1 Example of correct and incorrect paraphrasing

Angry Father. I'm so mad at my daughter that I could just wring her neck!"

Incorrect paraphrase: "You want to murder your daughter."

Correct paraphrase: "You are *really* furious with her!"

If you have, in the second example, accurately paraphrased the meaning of the angry father's intention, you will naturally go on to the next layer of his complaint.

Angry **Father.** "You won't believe what she did. I come home and find her on the couch lip-locking that punk from down the street. You know, the kid who epoxies his hair in corkscrew spikes?"

If, however, the second example is *inaccurate*, the angry father will correct you with more vehemence.

Angry Father. "No, not 'really furious.' I honestly intend to loop a belt around her neck and slowly strangle her. Seriously! She better not come home tonight."

At which point you will call law enforcement.

Why not Simply Ask the Person What Is Going On? If They Want to Tell Me, Why Don't They Just Answer the Questions?

We are aware that there are times that firefighters or EMTs <u>must </u>ask questions. There are medical emergencies that require immediate answers. Beyond that kind of immediate situation where every second counts, asking questions is usually not a good idea with really angry people. They already believe you have to 'get' what they're saying, and a question shows that you don't. The angry brain, focused on dominance hierarchy, sees your lack of comprehension as a deliberate act—an attack, in essence—on your part. Either you don't care to understand them, or your lack of understanding implies you find them to stupid to comprehend. Still angry and now frustrated at their failure, this makes them try harder, albeit with less organization and coherence than before. Over and over, they experience failure—they can't get through to you! When anger is combined with a sense of powerlessness, the person feels like he/she is 'losing' to a more powerful other. In essence, they experience a question, a demand for an answer, as putting you in a dominant position in regard to them.

Figure 45.2 Example of how irritating questions can be

Imagine coming home after a bad day. You're hot, tired, and frustrated. You walk into your house, drop your gear on the floor, sigh loudly, and walk toward the shower. Your spouse says, "Did you have a bad day?" Isn't this irritating? Isn't it *obvious* you've had a bad day? After all these years together, and he/she doesn't know when a bad day just walked into the house! On the other hand, imagine your spouse observing you and saying, "Bad day, huh?" You continue walking towards the shower, and say, "I don't want to talk now. I just want a shower. I'll talk to you later." You aren't 'forced' to explain yourself.

How to Use Paraphrasing Successfully

- It is very important that your voice is strong. You speak to the patient as someone who has the power within to take care of himself/herself and their problem, not as someone who is only fragile or volatile (even if he/she is at this moment).
- You must contact the strong aspect of the patient, the future looking side, that which is striving for integrity. If you contact the weak, or the insecure, you may foster regression to a less mature level of action. Childish action is often impulsive or violent. You are summing up your understanding, NOT comforting or providing emergency psychotherapy.
- Sometimes, you can use a dramatic summation, "You're really ticked off!" Here you sum up the patient's mood with your voice and posture, in addition to what is being said.

Using Paraphrasing to Communicate with Severely Mentally Ill Patients

Paraphrasing can be remarkably effective for communication with severely mentally ill patients. Given the internal chaos that people experience when psychotic, manic or disorganized, it is essential that we don't add to their sense of confusion by barraging them with questions or attempting to solve their problems by taking over and telling them what they should feel or do.

Figure 45.3 Example #1 of tactical paraphrasing with a psychotic patient

FIREFIGHTER/EMTs are called out to Murray's home, and find him in a decompensated state. Disheveled and staring in the first responders' direction, he says, "There are pink rose petals, rose petals flying all around my head, clouds and clouds of roses!"

One of the firefighters or EMT could ask him lots of questions in order to have him explain what he meant, but instead, he paraphrases the only thing he does grasp. (Notice the progression from one layer to another).

- **FIREFIGHTER/EMT**. "Pretty confusing, huh?"
- **Murray.** "You're darn right it's confusing. How'd you like to be in my head?"
- **FIREFIGHTER/EMT.** "I wouldn't want to be in a confused head. It must be hard to think."

- **Murray.** "Hard to think and scary. The roses turn bloody red, and I fly apart."
- **FIREFIGHTER/EMT.** "You can't keep things together."
- **Murray.** *(nodding)* "In the fear, it feels like blood."
- **FIREFIGHTER/EMT.** "Feels like blood, huh? I don't see any blood out here though."
- **Murray.** "In my head, only. Where the fear is."

Notice the responder's last sentence. Realizing that they have reached a 'core point' of Murray's concern, he intervenes more actively to validate his perception ("I don't see any blood out here, though…") and, at the same time, base him in reality. If, near the end, the firefighter or EMT had asked, "Is anybody hurt?" Murray might have been overwhelmed. Murray might think that the first responder seemed worried, and he could start thinking of all the people whose feelings he has hurt over the years, and wondering if he hurt someone and can't remember, etc. By making a matter-of-fact statement, the firefighter or EMT takes a lot of psychological pressure off him, and it is easier to re-organize enough to be able to communicate.

Remember, though, that paraphrasing is self-correcting. Murray might have replied, "There's no blood out here. She's lying in the back. That's where the blood is."

Figure 45.4 Example #2 of tactical paraphrasing with a manic patient

Johnny. "I never get enough sleep."

FIREFIGHTER/EMT. "You look really tired."

Johnny. "I don't know how I look, but I feel exhausted!"

When you're inaccurate in your summation, the other usually corrects you. He isn't arguing with you, just tuning up the signal.

FIREFIGHTER/EMT. "You've been up late the last couple days, waking early, and now you're really tired, aren't you?"

You can include extra information that sums up the experience the other is having. This is for the purpose of steering the patient toward problem-solving while not giving advice. It also allows you to assess how responsive he is to you. In other words, if you add a little something, is he even able to hear it?

Johnny. "I'm not tired at night."

FIREFIGHTER/EMT. "You can't fall asleep when you go to bed, huh?"

Notice the tag lines like, "huh?" or "aren't you?" These are not really questions. They follow statements and give the other an <u>invitation</u> to correct you or give you more information.

Johnny. "I don't even bother going to bed. I just lie there looking at the ceiling if I do."

FIREFIGHTER/EMT. "It seems like a waste of time, and then you wake up early anyway. It'd be fine if you weren't tired."

The second sentence by the first responder is an attempt to sum up what he believes is Johnny's feelings about his sleep cycle. It is also another assessment—he offers Johnny something to agree with or correct.

Johnny. "Yeah, I'd be fine if I wasn't tired. I'd just sleepless and do more. But I'm too tired for that. I wonder if I need to talk to Dr. Montour about my medications. I think I need something to help me sleep."

Imagine that Johnny is a young man who is very resistant to talking about his medications and one who usually gets in lots of trouble when he doesn't take them. If the first responder had responded to his initial statement about being tired by suggesting he go to the doctor immediately ('problem-solving'), Johnny might have angrily stopped talking or argued with him. By listening and showing step-by-step that he understood him, the first responder got Johnny to find the 'deeper layer' of his concern by himself.

Core

We know we have reached the core level when there is no more 'progress.' The person *spins his wheels*. They may use different words, but they say essentially the same thing over and over again. Some express relief at being finally understood. Some exhibit an intensification of emotion, because you have reached that which is most distressing. When you reach core, and it is clear that you're on the same wavelength, you can begin problem-solving. This can be:

- Further paraphrasing, where you show greater and greater understanding about what they're upset about.
- A summation of the core problem, followed by a puzzled "why?" For example, "You said you wanted to get better, but you checked yourself out of the hospital two nights ago, and you stopped taking your meds. So why didn't you follow your doctor's orders?"
- With some patients, you have, by paraphrasing them every step of the way, established that you're a person of trust. In some cases, you can now be quite directive, because people are often willing to accept advice or even instruction from those they trust.
- With others, we're ready to engage in a collaborative process of problem-solving, trying to figure out a way to solve the situation that is in the best interest of everyone involved.

Don't Waste It

Paraphrasing is almost a cliché, so much so that we can imagine some of you rolling your eyes when you read the title of this chapter. This technique is too important to abandon, and at the same time, it must be used carefully, i.e., *rarely*. If mentally ill contacts are used to your using paraphrasing as your primary method of discourse, they will cut you off, because you will appear to them to be giving nothing back, except mirroring. If the patient isn't angry and <u>requiring</u> you to use de-escalation tactics, don't use paraphrasing. Simply talk with them.

If there is a crisis, however, and the person doesn't believe they're understood, <u>now</u> paraphrasing comes into its own. Paraphrasing can have an almost electrifying effect with an angry patient. Imagine the feeling when you try to pull a splinter from under your fingernail, and after 10 long minutes of aggravating struggle, you get a hold of it finally and pull it out of your nail bed. That is the sense you get when, angry and desperate to be heard, you realize that the other person 'got it.'

Figure 45.5 How to master paraphrasing

As you as you view paraphrasing as a 'specialized,' pseudo-counseling technique, you probably won't want to do it—and you won't be good at it anyway. When you are hit by adrenaline, you will stumble over your words if you try to remember to say things like:
- "So what you are sharing with me is . . ."
- "What I hear you saying is . . ."

Don't do this! Many patients will find you irritating, and you will be in your head at a time where you must be aware of what's going on in front of you.

You are, in fact, a master of paraphrasing. You do it all the time simply keeping a conversation going, saying things like:
- "Your kid flunked out, huh?"
- "You're not getting a raise."
- "You hate that guy."
- "She's the one."

In short, the natural statements you intersperse in any conversation are perfect paraphrasing. However, because you do this unconsciously, it's hard to tap into as an *emergency technique.* It's easy to perfect, however. Consider this—how many conversations do you have a day? Twenty? Thirty? In each and every conversation, at an arbitrary moment of your choosing, decide to paraphrase the next thing they say. Just once. They won't even notice. But because you made a conscious decision to do this, <u>your brain notices</u>. That means you have practiced that skill twenty to forty times a day. Consider how good your tourniquet skills would be if you do twenty repetitions a day—it will be automatic! Similarly, if you do this every day, you will be able to step into crisis oriented paraphrasing without hesitation. It will be so natural to you that you do not even have to think about it.

CHAPTER 46

Some Guidelines
For Limit Setting

As soon as you draw a line it will become the main focus of your interchange. Don't ever set a limit that you can't enforce or one that isn't reasonable and simple to understand. When dealing with the mentally ill, <u>proper</u> limit setting is a kindness rather than oppression. Beleaguered by mental illness, struggling with substance abuse, beaten down by poverty or unemployment, such people experience their lives fragmenting into pieces. When the rules shift, they can become profoundly anxious. Limit setting helps them know where they stand.

Your tone of voice should be matter-of-fact. You shouldn't scold or criticize them. Simply remind them of the rule or set a proper limit (a new rule, so to speak). Only set reasonable limits that the person can do. If you can't explain clearly why the limit is necessary—at least to your peers—then it's not a good limit.

Setting a "Full Stop" Limit
- **Give clear directives with no wiggle room.** For example, you say in a confident, commanding voice, "Billy Jo, lower your voice. I can't attend to your wound."
- **If he complies, give him a brief mark of approval**. Continue with the verbal control.
- **If he doesn't comply with the directive, depersonalize the reiteration.** "Billy Jo, you are required to lower your voice." DON'T say, "I expect you to…." The patient should experience what you're saying as the 'law,' an institutional command or policy, rather than a personal issue between you both.
- **Don't get then caught up in manipulative word games.** Don't respond to professed ignorance, excuses or confusion. You're using this tactic because there is no ambiguity regarding the transgression and no ambiguity what the consequence will be.
- **Consequences.** "If you don't immediately stop yelling and threatening, then we will call law enforcement and you can work things out with them. You do understand that in the interim, you will be without medical care."
- **The 'choice.'** This follows almost directly from the previous step. With a detached tone, you will say, something like, "It looks like you've got a decision to make. But if you choose not to lower your voice, you know what will happen." You will follow through on your end based on whether they comply or not.
- **If they escalate.** If they simply escalate further, follow through as you promised.

CHAPTER 47

Techniques That Don't Work—
The Big Mistakes That Seemed
Like Such Good Ideas

Many of our mistakes are very obvious. As something leaves our mouth, we think, "Uh-oh. I shouldn't have said that!" But some are subtler, and often occur when we think we're doing the right thing.

Don't try to ingratiate yourself with the patient or try to pretend that the aggression isn't happening. Some firefighters and EMTs let the patient ramp up, but they try to tell themselves and others that they're letting them get it out of their system as a control tactic. In short, they cover their eyes and hope for the best. One of the paradoxes of ingratiation is that people who sell out their integrity often present themselves as having a 'special rapport' with the patient who, in fact, scares them.

The mistake of mind reading—taking a walk in someone else's head. Sometimes we try to steer people in the direction we want them to go by telling them either what we believe they are 'at heart,' or telling them what we (to be honest) wish they were. People may get quite offended by this, because it feels like you're claiming to read their minds. Statements like, "I know you really love your son," or "You don't really want to get into it with your neighbor," are statements that the angry person may not feel at all. When you make such generalized statements, people may feel compelled to prove you wrong by doing or saying exactly the opposite. If you do want to say something positive, praise a specific action and say it like this, "I know you're really mad, so I respect how you're keeping it under control and not going after him." And of course, only praise them for something that is true.

Getting it out of their system: The mistake of allowing venting. Pure venting is an expression of energy, such as going for a run after a difficult day, or chopping wood until fatigued, so that you can let go of a nasty incident at work. However, we also call generalized aggression expressed in front of others (tantrums), or aggression expressed about one person to another as venting.

Many people have a false idea about aggression. They imagine it to be some kind of psychological fluid that builds up pressure inside of us. These people believe that through venting, we get rid of the anger and then become peaceful. Aggression, however, isn't a fluid: it is an arousal state, and just like any other state of arousal—sexuality, happiness, excited interest—stimulus elicits more arousal. When we shout, yell, complain, kick things, or the like, we're escalating ourselves to greater and greater aggression. The longer you let aggression continue, the more generally 'aroused' the aggressor will be, and the harder it will be to control them.

When you let the potential aggressor vent about other people, it seems to them that you're giving covert approval to their complaints and verbal abuse. They believe you're on their side. When they're so angry that they start to become dangerous, and you *finally* object, they turn on you, feeling betrayed. Don't try to 'help them get it out of their system.' It doesn't work.

Head nodding. In Western culture, we generally nod our head once or twice followed by an interval of immobility when we're listening to another person. If we nod our head more than twice, in rapid succession particularly, this means we aren't interested and wish the person would be silent.

In some cultures, Japan being a prominent example, rapid and almost continuous head nodding and brief interjections like, "really, really, imagine that, yes, yes…." denote interest. In other cultures, nodding while someone is talking is considered rude, and people will, instead, hold their head still and look directly at you as a sign of respect. It is examples like these that illustrate the necessity of 'cultural information training.' Nonetheless, if you wish to be understood as listening with interest to someone in mainstream cultures, nod once or twice, and pause a long moment before nodding again.

Other really obvious mistakes that we shouldn't do, but we do anyway. *Don't!*
- Make promises you can't or don't keep. This will be experienced as betrayal.
- Make threats or promise consequences you can't keep. You will be viewed with contempt.
- Bombard the patient with choices, questions, and solutions. You will overwhelm them.
- Ask "Why?" to an angry or enraged person. There is usually no more unanswerable question, particularly when you're asking why someone is doing something. A 'why' question demands that the person 'explain himself/herself,' something they may be quite unwilling or even unable to do. (NOTE: the 'why' question when you've hit the core problem after a sequence of paraphrasing is the exception to this).
- Talk down to people as if they're stupid. This can be done, deliberately or inadvertently, when using unfamiliar vocabulary, jargon, or acronyms. It is also done when one sighs while the other is speaking, rolls one's eyes in contempt, or speaks slowly, as if talking to an idiot.
- Use global phrases like "Calm down." Specific commands get results. General commands don't.
- Analyze why they do something. Analyzing is 'cutting apart to examine.' People, upset or angry people in particular, experience being analyzed as a violation.
- Take it personally when they get upset.
- Interrupt people as they speak, particularly if you're correcting what they're saying. On the other hand, interruption of aggressive verbalizations or pointless monologues when you've got to get essential medical information is the right thing to do.
- Ignore it when they trespass on your boundaries. When we allow others to trespass on us, we're, implicitly giving them permission. Any territory we give up is free to whoever chooses to occupy it.
- Suspend boundaries. If we become too familiar, we become 'friends.' Sharing personal information or not setting limits leads the patient to viewing the relationship between you as eye-to-eye and reciprocal. It is very difficult to accept authority—limit setting, directions, or commands—

from a friend or equal. Safety is enhanced when one enforces a strong, decent but real hierarchical relationship.

- Boss them around in a demeaning or authoritarian way, particularly in front of their peers. Authoritarian attitudes and behaviors are among the most common precipitants of assault by mentally ill patients.
- Expose their private information in front of others.

Figure 47 Concerning privacy

Warning: Be careful of 'curbside debriefing.' You may be talking about a patient, either professionally, or just blowing off steam with complaints, jokes, or the like, and another person, perhaps mentally ill, hears you. That you aren't talking about them is irrelevant. They think, "If they talk about that woman like that, they're probably talking about me in the same way. The thought of that EMT talking about my family with that smile on his face makes me want to tear his face off!"

SECTION IX

Managing Rage and Violence

CHAPTER 48

The Nature Of Rage

Rage and anger aren't merely different in degree. They're different modes of being, just as water, once past the boiling point, becomes steam. Angry people posture to establish dominance or to force compliance. If nothing else, their goal is to communicate how angry they are. Enraged people, on the other hand, are in a 'threshold' state, trying to unleash themselves from whatever is holding them back from the violence they desire to commit. Therefore, all the strategies described in the previous section in dealing with the angry patient are more or less useless against the truly enraged. Let us note however, that we assigned anger arbitrarily within a scale of 20 to 95. This is a very broad range of arousal, ranging from mildly irritated to truly irate. Rage is 95 to 99, with a peak of 100 being violence. Taking into account, then, that these numbers are images rather than scientific measurements, we still may use some of the de-escalation strategies for anger when, for instance, the angry patient is at "93." For example, we have both used the tactic of "Breaking the Pattern" (Chapter 44) at just these moments, saying something so unexpected that it 'lets the air out of their tires.'

Past a certain point, however, the enraged patient is intent on committing mayhem. They only focus on how to overcome what is holding them back: fear of consequences, damage to their self-image, or innate morality. Their internal restraints are 'fighting' a battle within themselves against their primitive desire to maim and destroy.

There are various types of rage. It is very important to recognize what type of rage the aggressor is expressing, because there are different strategies to deal with each type. At the same time, don't worry that you will have a lot to remember. Enraged people's behavior is quite obvious. After reading this section, you will easily be able to tell what type of rage people are in, and will therefore know the best strategies to control them. Finally, although it is true that a patient can manifest a combination of several modes of rage, one mode will predominate, and THAT will be reflected in their behavior.[30]

Figure 48 IMPORTANT CAUTION

Here, and in several other areas of this book, we have used animal symbols to aid in the understanding of various types of rage or other behavior. For example, we use the image of a leopard or a shark in describing predatory rage. These are thought devices, and are not intended to be used in either paperwork or communication to describe such patients. In our hypersensitive times, such a reference to a specific patient may be misconstrued as stigmatizing them as 'being an animal.' Nothing could be further than the truth—the images are to assist in understanding modes of behavior, not character. Nonetheless, such images should remain aids of understanding, not terms of reference.

CHAPTER 49

Chaotic Rage—A Consideration Of Rage Emerging From Various Disorganized States

Patients who go into a chaotic rage are usually suffering from a confusion of thoughts and perceptions. They're disoriented, often experiencing severe hallucinations, illusions, and/or delusional thinking. Chaotic rage is common as part of a variety of syndromes, typified by profound disorganization of cognitive and perceptual processes, including severe psychosis that has 'crossed over' into a delirium state, mania, drunkenness, intoxication of various drugs, drug withdrawal, severe developmental disability, senile dementia, and a variety of inflammations or lesions of the brain. Unlike a classic psychosis, the most salient characteristic is that it is almost impossible to establish *any* lines of communication with the person.

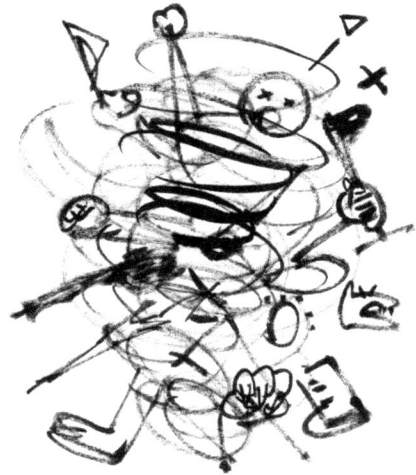

These patients often can't string their thoughts together logically; instead, they utter cascades of words making no sense whatsoever, or grunt, moan, or mumble. Others make sentences based on rhymes, puns, or cross-meanings, but with no calculation or plan. They may laugh or babble without any clear object, or completely out of proportion to the possible humor of the situation. The patient may speak in repetitive loops, becoming stuck on one subject, that could be real, hallucinatory, or so much a manifestation of their disorganization that you don't even know what they're talking about.

People in chaotic rage states can become quite frightened or irritable. They may begin yelling; screaming, lashing out physically, and engaging in such self-injurious acts as scratching and gouging their own flesh or head banging. Any state of chaotic rage should be considered a potential medical emergency that puts others as well as the patient at risk. De-escalation or control, in whatever form it takes, must be followed by medical attention as soon as possible. The delirium state, in particular, can be a sign of a life-threatening emergency.

Disorganized patients enter into chaotic rage states when they're frustrated, confused (too much stimulation), or feel invaded (for example, when you must carry out a necessary task, like physical assessment or transporting them to a hospital). Sometimes it is internally drive—a outcome of severe psychosis, a brain damaged by years of drug abuse, or an inordinate reaction to such drugs as PCP, 'bath salts' (cathinones) or Spice (synthetic cannabinoids). They can be simultaneously enraged and terribly frightened. Impulsive and unpredictable, their rage sometimes explodes, seemingly out of nowhere. Think of TAZ, the cartoon character in the Bugs Bunny cartoons.

People in a chaotic rage may strike out in all direction; they are often flailing and uncoordinated, but they're fully committed. What this means is that nothing—no fear of injury or consequences—holds them back from their attack. They may grab, scratch, bite, kick, and strike in flailing blows. They're often indifferent to or unaware of pain or injury to themselves. Some patients in chaotic rage actually target people to harm. Combat with them is like fighting a tornado of arms and legs. Others are so 'lost' that they aren't fighting, per se. They're 'swimming through people.' It is as if they're drowning, trying to struggle though a river, choked with wreckage, the people and objects around them the debris they're trying to swim through forcefully. However, some people in chaotic rage states, particularly trained fighters, retain their coordination even though they're completely 'gone' on a cognitive level. (In one infamous case in Washington State, a naked man in an excited delirium state still was able to pick up a police officer's dropped gun during their struggle, reinsert the magazine and shoot and kill the officer).

Figure 49.1 Example: 'coordinated' chaotic rage

One of the writers observed an elderly man with severe pugilistic dementia, coupled with alcohol intoxication—he knocked out two street punks who were harassing him with picture-perfect left and right hooks, then caught the bottle they had stolen in mid-air. Yet he could not articulate a coherent sentence.

De-Escalation of Chaotic Rage

Figure 49.2 Be patient—but never let down your guard

Some first responders, be they firefighters, EMTs or police get impatient watching another first responder take their time to get the disorganized person under control through verbal tactics. Just as the lead EMT or firefighter is achieving verbal control, an impatient member of the crew jumps in, and then all hell breaks loose.

Nonetheless, disorganized patients are among the most difficult to de-escalate verbally because words and coherent cognitive processes are the first things that they lose. You must, therefore, be prepared to evade a sudden attack, and further, be prepared, **throughout**, to use physical control tactics to ensure your safety as well as that of others (Chapter 7).

- Disorganized people are both impulsive and unpredictable. Therefore, knowledge of any triggers that might have set them off in the past is essential.
- Use calm movements, and a firm but reassuring voice. Delirious people often experience poor motor control, experienced as vertigo, disorientation, etc. Your voice and slow movements helps them orient, not only physically, but as an emotional touchstone as well.

- Disorganized people are susceptible to being deflected to another topic. They often use *confabulation*, the concoction of spurious memories, as a means of trying to appear normal and stable. You can sometimes "confabulate" a theme yourself that catches their attention and seems to engage higher thought processes, delaying their outburst of rage until help can arrive.

Figure 49.3 Example of deflection when dealing with a person in a chaotic rage state

A paramedic approached a delirious man who was standing on the edge of a highway, and said, "Ike, what are you doing here. I haven't seen you since high school." As he kept rattling off spurious memories to the man, whose name *wasn't* Ike and whom he had never seen before, the delirious man gazed into his eyes in confusion, rocking back and forth in rhythm with the paramedic's words. The paramedic was successful in capturing the man's attention, which kept him from dashing into traffic, until police could arrive. To illustrate how dangerous this situation was, the moment the police tried to physically ease him back from the highway, the man exploded into a violent attack, requiring a number of cops to subdue him.

- One of the last things we 'retain' is our name, so use their name, repetitively, interspersing it frequently in your commands in order to get their attention before initiating attempts to redirect them to another activity. This can be very helpful with combat veterans experiencing a 'flashback.'[31]
- Be very cautious about touching them, as this may be experienced as invasive or even as an attack. If you do have to lay hands on them, make sure you have enough hands and bodies to totally control them.
- As was described in detail in the chapter on disorganization (Chapter 22), use simple, concrete commands with no more than a single 'subject' in each sentence. Repetition several times is almost always helpful. Use only one thought at a time, as complex sentences will be confusing, and thus threatening or irritating. For example, say *slowly*, "Sit down, William. Sit down. Sit down. William, sit down."
- Minimize such distracting behaviors on your part as extraneous body movements. Your movements should be calming and also only be those useful in helping the person understand what is going on.
- Be cognizant of the volume on your radio. It can be very distracting and it may overshadow what either of you is saying.
- Use tactical paraphrasing (Chapter 45), summing up apparent mood, not specific ideas or life circumstances. You can sometimes help by validating and acknowledging their confusion or fear. For example, "Really scary, huh?" or "You're really worried, aren't you?"
- Because of their difficulty in attending to what you say, non-verbal communication is a paramount concern. A calm reassuring presence, manifesting both strength and assurance is your best hope of helping to stabilize a patient in chaotic rage.

Excited Delirium Syndrome

Excited delirium (Appendix C for a state-of-the-art protocol for response to this syndrome) is a rare condition at the extreme end of the hyper-aroused wing of chaotic rage. Etiology can be varied, but it is most commonly associated with long-term use of stimulants—particularly cocaine and methamphetamine—and sometimes single dose episodes or binges of phencyclidine (PCP), 'bath salts' (cathinones), Spice (synthetic cannabinoids) and on rare occasions, psychedelic drugs, such as LSD or psilocybin mushrooms. It is also associated with extreme manic or psychotic excitement, and can be precipitated by a variety of purely medical conditions. It is typified by some, if not all of the following:

- a sudden onset of extreme agitation
- pervasive terror, often without object
- chaotic, sudden shifts in emotions and disorientation
- screaming, pressured incoherent speech, grunting, and irrational statements
- aggression to inanimate objects, particularly shiny objects like glass and mirrors
- hyper-arousal with unbelievable strength, endurance, and insensitivity to pain
- hyperthermia accompanied by stripping off clothes
- violent resistance to others <u>before, during, and after</u> arrest or restraint.

Accompanying their almost unbelievable level of physical arousal and resistance to both physical and mechanical restraints is possible respiratory and cardiac arrest. **These people die!** The usual pattern is that they struggle with incredible power, and then they suddenly stop moving. Or sometime after becoming quiet, either in a stupor or in seeming normality, they die, usually from cardiac arrest. This can look remarkably similar to a seizure, also a very dangerous syndrome.

Correct protocol demands that EMS and police are called simultaneously, and that EMS should ready to intervene medically the *instant* the patient is physically subdued. Such patients can be appallingly dangerous both to others and to themselves. *We can't emphasize strongly enough that this is a medical emergency manifesting as physical danger, and usually requiring both police and emergency medical intervention to secure the person so that they can be treated. The EMTs or paramedics need to be prepared to treat a cardiac arrest situation.*

You will, almost surely, be unable to verbally de-escalate the person in excited delirium, but if they aren't presenting an immediate assault risk, make the attempt using the principles delineated above, particularly repetitive commands at a regular, slow cadence (Chapter 22). Delirious individuals sometimes 'flicker' in and out of full delirium states, and in the 'intervals,' you may be able to gain partial compliance that makes it easier to for the police (or in some circumstances, firefighters and EMTs) to place them in physical restraint, ideally and immediately followed by chemical restraint (Appendices A, B, C). If nothing else your verbal control tactics may 'buy time' allowing sufficient emergency personnel to muster, making possible the restraint that will most likely be necessary to get them help.

Figure 49.4 Excited delirium or chaotic rage

Most patients who go into chaotic rage aren't in an excited delirium, but given the ever-increasing abuse of stimulants (methamphetamine, cocaine, etc.) that are the most common precipitants of this condition, it is important that you are familiar with the signs, symptoms, and 'best-practice' interventions. Furthermore, we strongly urge local law enforcement, emergency rooms, paramedic organizations, and 9-1-1 dispatch centers to become fully familiar and trained to deal with patients suffering from this syndrome. A joint training of all responders who may be involved in the restraint and treatment of such patients is imperative. You need to have an established protocol to ensure public safety, first responder safety, and the safety, as best as you can accomplish it, of the delirious patient.

Greater knowledge about this syndrome has led to several new problems:

a. The protocol for Excited Delirium is to subdue the patient as quickly as possible to get them the medical attention they need, as well as protecting everyone from the appalling violence they may enact. As most mentally ill patients, including severely disorganized people, are NOT in excited delirium states, this protocol can seem to directly contradict the model of verbal de-escalation we have offered in this book. In brief, with most mentally ill patients, take extra time to talk them into compliance, but with patients manifesting excited delirium, they need to be subdued as quickly as possible. However, a careful reading of this text reveals a graduated set of interventions, including how to approach a disorganized patient, even one manifesting chaotic rage. As we have emphasized throughout the text, that assessment is behaviorally based, any dangerous behavior on the part of the person of concern should elicit a well-practiced physical response.

b. Because Excited Delirium has finally begun to be recognized by the medical community as a genuine medical syndrome, this complicates things for non-medical personnel. Psychosis, unlike schizophrenia, is a general term. Therefore, it is usable. However, if a firefighter or EMT uses the term Excited Delirium, he/she can be accused of diagnosing the person. Therefore, we recommend the use of the terms Chaotic Rage to describe such patients, both in paperwork and as part of your protocols and those of police and 9-1-1 dispatch. It is fully descriptive, encompassing both the disorganization AND the agitation that such patients display. Furthermore, the firefighter or EMT isn't required to make a distinction between a person with genuine excited delirium, a mushroom intoxicated naked man running down the street, or a distraught grief-stricken patient in a chaotic state. All responders, from police, corrections, fire, EMS, and dispatch can use this descriptive term without running the risk of being either over-specific or diagnosing in the street.

c. These terms will help firefighters and EMTs, on a behavioral basis, to distinguish Chaotic Rage from lower levels of disorganization or psychosis so that best practice interventions can be used.

d. Refer to the Appendix C for specific protocols for firefighters and EMT in dealing with Chaotic Rage

Catatonia: Special Considerations

People may be immobile for many reasons—among them being a variety of medical concerns. Catatonia however, is a very rare, very bizarre condition in which a patient stays in a fixed posture, not congruent with injury or seizure. Catatonia is caused either by mental illness (schizophrenia) or an organic condition: for example, drug toxicity. The catatonic person's posture may be quite awkward or twisted, seeming to require great flexibility. A classic symptom of true catatonia is 'waxy immobility,' whereby if someone else moves the catatonic's body or limbs, he/she maintains the posture into which they were moved. There seems to be no way to establish any communication link with them.

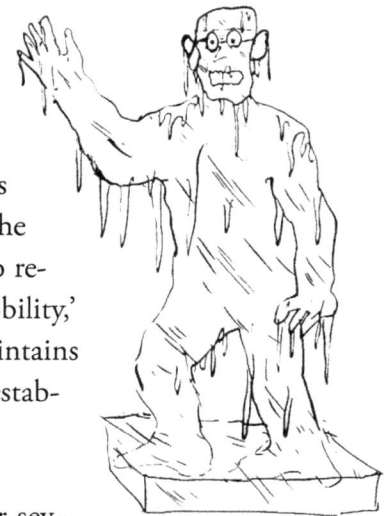

Considerable caution is needed in dealing with immobile patients for several reasons. First, they may be injured or having a seizure and at medical risk. For this reason a medical evaluation is *always* indicated. A second consideration is safety. One way to regard catatonia is to view the patient as exerting 100 percent of their resources to *not* interact with the outside world. You may be tempted to get them to respond when they're unsecured. This is a disastrous mistake. Image the incredible exertion of will required to maintain immobility for hours, even days: without movement, without response, without even blinking in some cases. Now imagine disturbing this equilibrium. The result is what is clinically called 'catatonic rage,' a state that really can be considered one form of excited delirium (above). The patient shifts from 100 percent stillness to 100 percent explosive motion. One of the authors can recall an incident where a police officer's career was ended by such a patient who, all of 110 pounds, suddenly 'woke up' and grabbed hold of his arm and yanked as if he was cracking a whip, ripping through all the ligaments of the officer's shoulder and shoulder blade.

You would be wrong to think the catatonic is unaware; they *can* hear you. Therefore, speak calmly and respectfully. A patient can have a very long memory of being shamed, and if you speak about or treat the catatonic as an object rather than as a person, you may evoke a terrible sense of humiliation. In their frozen state, they may not be able to do anything about it now, but months or years later, someone who resembles the person who humiliated them may be the object of that postponed rage. Another firefighter or EMT may be hurt, having no idea that the mentally ill person they're dealing with has been waiting for years for an opportunity to avenge his/her humiliation. Beyond all that, everyone—even a person in a coma—deserves to be treated with respect. Even if it seems that the catatonic person can't hear a word that you're saying, act as if they're listening to every word.

If you have any suspicion that a patient may be catatonic, place them in restraints and transport them to a hospital where they can be evaluated safely. Do everything in your power to ensure that police assist you in smoothly moving the patient onto a gurney and into restraints with a minimum of jostling, loud voices or cross-talk. Testing reactivity to pain, light or noise, for example, shouldn't occur until the patient is safely in restraints. When you move them to a gurney, make sure you have sufficient numbers to safely manage them, just in case they were to explode suddenly while being moved.

De-escalation of Developmentally Disabled Patients: Special Considerations

De-escalation tactics aren't remarkably different with developmentally disabled folks, but one must be aware of their cognitive deficits. If you use language that is too sophisticated, either in terms of meaning or nuance, you may elicit more frustration and anger, because you will be making them 'feel stupid.'

Many developmentally disabled people are subject to 'magical thinking.' Their beliefs about the material world and their own powers and vulnerability often don't conform to reality. Sometimes one can use these beliefs to help calm them, as you would with a child. On other occasions, one must be aware of these beliefs to keep the situation from escalating out of control.

If you try to control a developmentally disabled patient based on their physical age (a 250 pound, 35-year-old adult, for example), things usually go very wrong very fast. Most of our associates have found that once we make eye-contact, we can estimate the emotional age of the developmentally disabled person very quickly. Speak to them at their emotional age: small child, young kid, or teen. This may seem very abstract, but it is really simple. You look in their eyes, and if you see a childish expression just like that of your own five year old, ten year old, or thirteen year old, interact with them at that level. If you don't 'catch' such an intuition, then just follow standard de-escalation procedures. To be very clear: Safety considerations are unchanged—what is different is the way you verbally interact with them.

Figure 49.5 Example of Incident With a Developmentally Disabled Patient

A developmentally disabled woman once grabbed my finger, trying to break it. I neutralized her attempt by shifting the angle of my hand as she yanked, and as she was at the emotional age of about 8 years-old, rather than commanding her to "let go!" I said, "I know you want to hold my hand. You don't have to twist my finger. We can hold hands as much as you like. Sure, we can hold hands." She suddenly let go and dropped to the floor, crying.

We're NOT asserting that things will always go well! One of the writers recalls another incident where an EMT tried to treat a 225 pound, 40 year-old man with a lacerated wrist, who was sitting quietly in one of the group home chairs. He talked with the man gently, at his emotional age of about eight or nine years old. As the EMT attempted to put pressure on the wound, without any warning, the patient slugged him in the head, then knocked another firefighter off her feet as well.

Don't let down your guard, just because the person does have a childlike presentation. You can talk to them at their age, without suspending, in the slightest, a combative mindset. There are many occasions when you can use tactical paraphrasing (Chapter 45) with an enraged developmentally disabled patient.

Don't just sum things up calmly. Use an almost dramatic voice, over-emphasizing words. "YOU'RE REALLLLLY upset. You're SO upset about this! I GOT IT!!!" Your voice is a combination of drama and enthusiasm. In essence, you're trying to catch their attention with charisma, a kind of energy in which you change the dynamics of your relationship through your voice and demeanor. The angry or enraged developmentally disabled aggressor finds himself/herself in an interaction where there is no 'fight' coming from you.

You can use the same communication style with a developmentally disabled patient (just as you would with a child) who is disappointed or unhappy. "Wow. You REALLY loved that book! I KNOW that. You really, really wanted to keep it!" Your dramatic voice validates how important the situation is to the person. It is the voice, here, more than the words that provide that validation.

Talking With a Disorganized Person After a Crisis

It can be tactically sound to validate feelings, both for yourself and for them, after a crisis, if they are cognitively intact at the moment to listen to you. Remember, though this is for the purpose of increasing your ability to control them—it isn't for the purpose of therapy! For example:

- "Marc that was really scary."
- "I'm glad that's over!"
- "I want you to sit on this chair now."
- "Yeah, I know you were scared."

A detailed critique of what they did, however, is a mistake. People who are disorganized are often cognitively impaired, and this affects their memory as well. Their feelings, also, aren't under their control, and they will react to your debriefing as if it is a new attack, especially if you put your feelings into what you say. Your primary concerns should be behavioral stability (no new attack) and reassurance, because they're very likely to be afraid that you may want to get back at them.

CHAPTER 50

Terrified Rage

Figure 50.1 Concerning Terrified Rage and Chaotic Rage

Be aware that the line between terrified rage and chaotic rage can be very fine. The terrified person, overwhelmed, can shift into chaotic rage. When facing a patient in a state of either pure terror or terrified rage, be prepared, therefore, to shift to protocols suitable to assisting patients in chaotic states when necessary (Chapter 49).

Terrified patients believe that they will be violated or abused. They look halfway ready to run, halfway ready to strike. Their voice can be pleading, whiny, or fearful, and their eyes are often wide-open or darting from place to place.

The mouth of a terrified person often gapes slightly as they breathe in panicky, short gasps. Other frightened people press their lips together in a quivering pucker. Their breathing is often panicky, fast and high in the chest. Their skin tone is often ashen or pale. They make threat gestures with a flailing overhand blow or a fending off gesture. Their body posture is concave, pulling away from you as much as possible. They may cower or crouch.

Figure 50.2 Caution—Wide open eyes does not always indicate terror

Wide-open eyes doesn't always indicate fear. In the case of fear, the muscles under the eyes are also slack, giving the face a pleading look. Even though the terrified person may be looking in your direction, they usually don't look *into* your eyes, nor do they want you to look into theirs. The enraged, aggressive patient with wide-open eyes, on the other hand, displays tension around the eyes. Furthermore, they often look penetratingly into your eyes, or *through* you.

When they yell, there is a hollow quality, as if their voice has no foundation. This is due to the tightening of their abdomen and diaphragm, so that not only their breathing, but also their speech, is high in their chest.

There is usually high physical arousal, accompanied by panting, sweating, and trembling. They often back into a wall or corner. Their body is usually tense, preparing to either defend or flee. They may yell, almost screaming in a pleading tone, such phrases as: "Stay back!" "You get away from me!" "I will hit you!! I will!" "You stay back!"

What Causes Terrified Rage?

People who are terrified often suffer from paranoid delusions, a fear of the unknown, or terrifying hallucinations. At other times, they're afraid of a loss of control, or of being laughed at or humiliated. Some people are afraid that they're in terrible trouble with some agency, be it the police or medical/mental health personnel. Finally, for any one of a number of reasons, they're simply terrified of you.

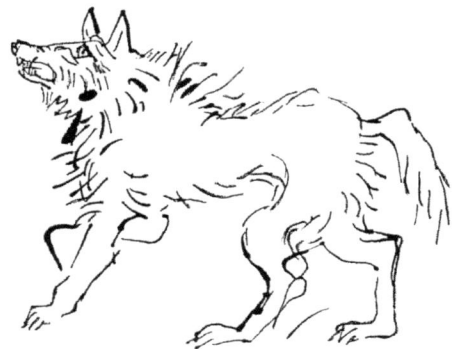

De-Escalation of Terrified Rage

Imagine a snarling wolf cornered, backed up against a cliff face. It is a frightened animal with fangs—do you think that what it really needs right now is a hug? Your goal is to reduce their sense of danger. Move away from them, slowly. Relax your posture. Make sure your movements are unhurried. Your voice is firm, confident, and reassuring.

Notice if their body relaxes or tenses in response to your eye contact. If eye contact is reassuring for the patient, signified by a more relaxed posture, do so; if intimidating, don't. Keep looking in their direction, of course.

Keep up a reassuring litany of phrases, speaking slowly, with pauses: "I know you're scared--that's okay.------Put down the chair.--------You don't need that.--------I keep it safe here. You can put it down now.-------I'm way over here.------Go ahead. Sit down. I keep it safe."

DON'T say, "I'll protect you" or "I won't hurt you." Many people who go into terrified rage have a history of victimization and have been hurt before by people who said those kinds of phrases. However, when you say, "I keep it safe here," you're being the alpha who says, "This is my territory and no one, including you, will be hurt on my territory. I'm taking responsibility now—through me and because of me, this place and you in it—will be safe." Furthermore, by saying something similar to what they expect to hear, but somehow different, you cause a 'glitch' in their thought process. The frightened person thinks: "What did he say? He didn't say, 'I won't hurt you.' What's different in what he said?" By getting the terrified person *questioning* what you said, you cause him to 're-engage' the parts of his brain that actually thinks things through as opposed to just reacting.

You will easily be able to observe it in their body language as they calm down. Their breathing will get a little shuddery or be expressed in short high-pitched gasps. Often they will slump into a chair or the floor and even begin to weep. Keep up with your reassuring litany, and approach them slowly. If they show signs of getting frightened again, pause, move back slightly, and continue to speak to them reassuringly.

When you approach, move in 'half-steps.' Move the right foot a full step, then bring the left foot *up* to the right foot. Pause. Move either right or left foot forward, and then bring the other foot forward *up* to the lead foot. Pause and then continue. The advantage of moving this way is that you stay balanced, in case the patient attacks suddenly: you don't have too much forward momentum. Additionally, if the person becomes *more* startled or reactive, you can ease backward smoothly, creating more space between you. When you walk normally, one foot in front of the other, changing directions is more 'dramatic.' You have to make a big movement, maybe even lurching backwards, and this action can contribute to an *increase* in the terrified person's agitation.

CHAPTER 51

Hot Rage

When we think of people on the edge of violence, it is hot rage that usually comes to mind. We imagine ourselves faced with someone with muscles writhing, yelling, or screaming, fist brandished and threatening. They throw things, tip over desks, and spit in our face. They want to beat us bloody, stab us, or pound us into a pulp.

We often imagine that hot rage is instinctual, a product of primitive drives: a reflex. However, purely instinctual aggression is uncoordinated and flailing: such rage falls under the category of terrorized or chaotic aggression. Hot rage, however, is coordinated. This makes it a behavior that is learned through modeling, trained through repetition, and reinforced through success. Therefore, it could be referred to as a 'pseudo-instinct,' a trained response that functions reflexively.

For example, some people with a long history of abuse lash out in rage whenever frightened, with no ability to evaluate whether or not they're currently in danger. At the same time, they target where best to hit, and frequently choose a time and a place where they believe they have the best chance of success. On a more functional level, a good street fighter, even though he has 'lost it,' still takes a stance with chin tucked in, shoulder rolled forward, and punches with his entire body lined up, so that the power of the blow is amplified by his body weight and the torque of his hips.

Some claim that hot-rage is an expression of extreme frustration, but frustration alone doesn't usually elicit rage in normal people. It is when frustrated desires are coupled with something 'personal'—when one believes oneself to be *impeded* by another person in getting one's desires met—that he or she becomes enraged. In other words, the enraged person believes that they are right and justified to become violent. There are three subtypes of hot rage: Fury, Bluffing, and Aggressive-Manipulation.

General information About Hot Rage
- This mode is typified by emotional arousal or excitement.
- Bored people with aggressive tendencies, bullies, or others who simply need a lot of nervous energy to feel alive will amp up aggression to feel this energy and power.
- Over-arousal leads to a deterioration in judgment, and at higher states of arousal, even deterioration of basic cognitive processes.

Figure 51.1 Example of Hot Rage Escalating Into Violence

A man is walking down the street and sees a father slap his child's face. He intervenes, saying, "That's just a child. Be easy on him." The angry father shoves him and says, "Mind your own business, or I'll give it to you, too."

The man later describes hearing a high pitched noise, and his vision turning black-and-white. He comes to himself astride the abusive man, pounding his face with his fists.

- Arousal breeds arousal. The more enraged people become, the more comfortable they're with their rage, and the easier it becomes to be violent.
- Hot rage is often a behavior that has led to short-term success in the past, such as scaring and beating a selected victim either for criminal gain, or just for the joy of it. In a state of rage, such a person has no concern about longer-term consequences, much less guilt.
- For some people, there is a sense of liberation, even a paradoxical kind of joy when they peak into rage. All one's fears and insecurities disappear, and one is left with only the ecstasy of the pure act. Some patients desire rage, because that ecstatic state is, to them, the best thing they ever feel.
- Displacement is common: Instead of hitting you (yet), they first hit an available target like a chair, wall, or other objects. This also includes picking things up and slamming them down, or throwing things. Predatory individuals (Chapter 52) also use displacement as a tactic to make their target more fearful. Those in a state of hot rage are simultaneously terrorizing their target, discharging tension and, and at the same time, 'warming up' to attack.
- Hot rage can be a 'transference' in which the first responder is a stand-in for someone else. In their mind, you're the emblem of everyone who ever controlled them or put them down, an agent of an oppressive society, or simply a legitimate target to express hatred and violence.
- There can also be organic contributors: low blood sugar levels, head injury, or the use of intoxicants that lessen the patient's inhibitions.
- Hot rage is also associated with peer group influence and masculine display: 'fronting' in front of one's group. It can have a resonating effect among such a group, creating mob violence, one person's rage fueling another.

De-Escalation of Hot Rage: The Ladder

The primary method of de-escalation for hot rage is called 'The Ladder.' It is used only for rage, that gray zone between anger (even extreme anger) and violence. The patient is no longer trying to communicate with you. They're right on the edge of assault—in a sense, doing a war dance to work out inhibitions to committing violence. Don't hold back from any action to keep yourself and others safe. Protect yourself and/or others! Verbal control is, of course, ideal with people in a state of rage, but if they cross the line into violence, do what you have to do to stay safe.

The technique itself is simple. Use a short sentence with no more than four or five words. Choose the most dangerous behavior and repetitively command that it cease. Use short words. (Don't use 'psychologese,' like "It's not appropriate for you to…..") Once dangerous behavior stops, choose the next level down of problematic behavior and use the same technique. Continue until the patient is de-escalated and under control. This technique is only effective right before, during, and after the peak of the crisis because it is a 'Control Tactic' rather than the 'Lining Up' that we use for angry people. Control tactics will provoke rage in an angry person, someone we might have over-estimated, due to his/her loud tone, or dramatic behaviors. As described earlier, facing an enraged person causes us to experience fear in a way that anger does not. Remember the image of the spider (Chapter 37): Is it in the box or out on the floor? If the person is in a rage state, the danger is NOW, not merely something possible if the situation continues to deteriorate

With the ladder technique, you establish a hierarchy of danger. What you need to perceive is what action of the enraged person is most dangerous or problematic. The general hierarchy from most to least is as follows:
1. Brandishing an object as a weapon or a weapon itself in a menacing way. (NOTE: If they're too close, or are trying to use the weapon, this is a situation of violence, not rage). All force options should be considered.
2. Approaching or standing too close to you with menacing intent.
3. Kicking objects, punching walls, or throwing things (displacement activity).
4. Pacing, stomping, and inflating the body in an aggressive manner (posturing).
5. Shouting, or talking in low, menacing tones.
6. Using language that is intended to violate, demean, or degrade.

Give the aggressor a straightforward command to stop their most dangerous behavior. You shouldn't scream or shout—that won't get through to the person. Instead, they will ramp up on your screaming tone, and this, alone will increase their aggressive energy. Rather, your voice should be strong, low and commanding (Chapter 42).

This isn't the time to be trying to think of something brilliant or life changing to say. By keeping things simple, you use your mind to keep track of your crew, other potential aggressors, escape routes, and where weapons might be. In addition, by holding to a demand that the most dangerous behavior cease, you are displaying clarity and strength to the aggressor, as well as helping them focus his/her mind on the most problematic thing he/she is doing. This is something particularly important with a mentally ill patient who may truly have lost it, and among other things, needs help orienting back to this world where it is so profoundly not-a-good-thing to assault first responders.

After a couple of repetitions, always add, "We'll talk about it when you…." This provides them with an 'out,' be it a face-saving opportunity, or a genuine alternative to what they were intending. Once that behavior is stopped, pick the next most problematic behavior, and command/require that it stops. If the aggressor does calm down and stops all the aggressive behaviors, including assaultive language, THEN set a firm and direct limit. You should frequently intersperse your sentences with their name, using this to pace and break the rhythm of your commands, as well as 'calling them back' to a human relationship, name to name.

The Ladder isn't merely a verbal intervention. Like any other control tactic with an aggressive patient, but particularly with hot rage, you must move as needed to maintain the optimum space to both defend yourself and exert maximum influence upon them. If they're very close, or threatening, depending on the situation, your hands should be:

- up in the fence position, prepared to fight as well as ward off any attack, but also as a gesture that is both calming and dominant;
- clasping the wrist of one hand with the other hand.

You continue to work your way down the "rungs" until the aggressor is no longer in a state of fury. If the patient re-escalates to a higher and more dangerous activity, simply go up to that 'rung' of the ladder and begin repeating again. Remember to stand and use your voice as described in the previous sections. Usually, the last rung is either shouting, or even further down—swearing and using demeaning, ugly language.

Figure 51.2 Example of the Ladder

Your voice is firm, low pitched and commanding, as you 'descend' down the rungs. You should imagine that there are pauses, sometime of several seconds or more, between each phrase below. In the following scenario, each statement is, of course, in response to something the aggressor has done or said. Don't talk too fast—a firm cadence shows strength.

1. "Step back. Step back. Robert. We'll talk about it when you step back. Robert. Step back. Step back, Robert. We will talk about it when you step back."
2. "Stop kicking things. Robert. Stop kicking things. We'll talk about it when you stop kicking things."
3. "Robert, I can't follow you when you pace around. Sit down and we can talk. Sit down, Robert."

Notice the paradoxical message, that you can't 'follow' him. Of course you could, if you wanted to. This is another example of what we call a 'brain glitch'" the same as we do with the patient in Terrified Rage, when we say, "I keep it safe here." You are trying to catch their attention as they try to make sense of what you said. We want them thinking again, trying to figure out what you said and why you said it. We want the part of the brain that thinks things through taking over from the part that is driving them towards violence.

Imagine they have stepped forward again, thus ascending to a higher 'rung' on the ladder

1. "Step back! Robert! Step back and we'll talk. We will TALK about it when you step back, Robert. Step—back."

2. "Sit down Robert. We will talk about it when you sit down. We can't talk when you are walking around. We will talk about it when you sit down."
3. "Lower your voice. I can't hear you when you yell that loud. Lower you voice and we will talk."

Here is a second paradoxical communication; of course, you can hear an aggressor who is shouting loudly. Once again, you are trying to create a 'glitch' where he tries to figure out what you mean when you say you can't hear him when he is yelling.

"Talk to me with the same respect that I talk to you. We will talk about it when you stop swearing. Stop swearing. Robert. We will talk when you talk to me with respect, the same way I talk to you."

Remember, people often swear as punctuation. They have no hostile intent whatsoever. If the patient is swearing in this manner, it isn't a problem. For example, "hey, I'm sorry, I was just mad at my f**king daughter, and s**t, you happened to arrive at just the wrong damn moment."

However, if the swearing is an attempt to violate you, it **must** *be dealt with in proper order. However,* **don't** *focus on the language, no matter how vile, if the aggressor is doing something dangerous. Remember that predatory patients will use language to shock, distract, immobilize or terrorize. What they're* **doing** *is far more dangerous than anything they're saying.*

Figure 51.3 Caution
Remember, the ladder should only be used with an enraged patient. Using this technique with an angry patient will cause them to escalate into rage. In most cases, de-escalation tactics suitable to dealing with angry patients are sufficient.

Figure 51.4 How about if they object that "you aren't talking to me yet."
Remember the face-saving phrase, "We'll talk about it when you . . .?" Sometimes the individual will say, "Wait a minute. You said we 'd talk about it when I stepped back, and THEN you said we'd talk about it when I stopped hitting things, and THEN you said we'd talk about it when I stood still. You are messing with me!"

Reply in the following manner. "Mr. Jackson, that's great! If you can pick up on that, that means your are ready to work this out instead of taking this in a dangerous direction. You are ready to talk with me? OK, then sit down, stop yelling and swearing and we will talk this out."
However, if he then continues to be threatening, or re-escalates, go 'back' to the ladder.

Hot Rage Subtype #1: Fury
Take control until the patient can achieve it on his own

What does fury look like? Furious people look as if they're about to explode. *If they're of big stature, think of a grizzly bear. If they're smaller, think of a wolverine.* In either case, the image suggests an animal that will tear you to pieces to get what it wants. Many people, with or without a mental health diagnosis, show hot rage. It is particularly common among people who have suffered head injuries. The following are physical manifestations of hot rage:

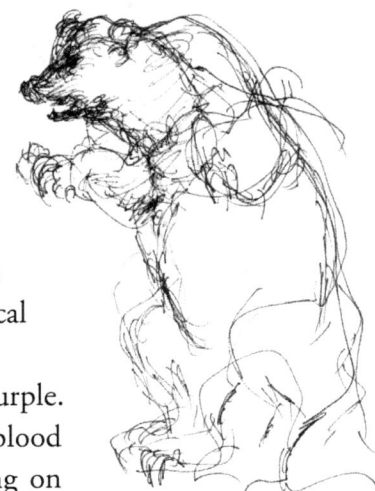

- Their skin tone is flushed as they're angered, becoming red or purple. As they become even more enraged their skin blanches, as the blood pools in the internal organs. They turn pale or gray, depending on whether their skin is light or dark.
- Their voice, be it loud, low and quiet, has a menacing and belligerent tone.
- They often pace, inflate their upper body, and hit things or smash their hands together, often one fist in the other hand.
- They tend to stare into your eyes directly. The eyes may be wide open, but definitely NOT in the same manner as the terrified person. There will be tension all around the eyes, and they stare directly into yours. Others glower, looking out under their brows. In either event the face is furious and hostile.
- Their eyes may appear red or inflamed.
- Physical arousal, blood pressure, and muscular tension all increase. You will sometimes see veins pop out of the skin, particularly around the neck.
- Sometimes they will have a smile that shows no humor or joy. Others snarl, or compress their lips with a twist, as if they have a foul taste in their mouth. Still others bare their teeth—sometimes edge-to-edge—or clench their jaws so tightly that the muscles stand out in bunches.
- They're very impulsive, and unconcerned with possible consequences.
- Depending on their emotions, which include how comfortable they're with the rage they're experiencing, their breathing is either strained or easy. The person usually breathes deeply from the chest into the belly. They often draw the belly inward on the inhale as their chest inflates.
- They may claim to be disrespected, humiliated, or shamed. Others will allege that they aren't getting their questions answered or their problem solved, or that no one listened or cared. They may rant about some person or system or claim that these are their enemy. This is often the pretext they use to amp themselves up into fury.
- At their most dangerous point, they may become calm, breaking off eye-contact, or go into a thousand-yard stare.

Control of Fury
- Your posture and tone should be confident, commanding, even imposing.
- Stand out of range of an immediate blow, but directly in front of them. If you're too close, it is

a challenge; too far away, you will be seen as afraid, and you will be a target to vent their frustration. You may have to move forward and back to maintain this spacing. Try to move smoothly, without flinching. When you move with a relaxed body, you're more ready to protect yourself, yet you don't appear as if you're trying to initiate a fight.

- Stand with your feet in a 'blade' stance, with one foot advanced, and the other behind at about a forty-five degree angle. (If you drew the back foot forward, there would be one or two fist's space between the heels—don't line-up the feet, one behind the other.) This best prepares you to slip along tangents to his attack, to ward off blows, or to fight back if necessary. Don't square your feet so that you're confronting him/her in full frontal fashion: not only are the most vulnerable areas of your body exposed to attack, you're 'flat-footed.' To avoid an attack or to fight back, you'll have to first shift your weight to one foot or the other before you can move. With the blade stance, you're already 'chambered' to do this.
- As described earlier, your hands are either up in a fence, or the wrist of one arm is clasped in the hand of the other in front of you at waist level.
- Your voice is strong and forceful. Don't, however, shout. Instead, keep your voice low- pitched and calm, dropping it into your chest where it resonates, as enraged people, in particular, react violently to threatening or angry vocal tones. The only time you should shout is a 'battle cry,' the lion's roar that you use only when you're trying to stop an actual attack.
- Use direct eye contact, and say their name frequently, interspersing it among your commands.
- Use the Ladder in its most orthodox form with your voice pitched low and powerful. You should feel it vibrate in your chest.

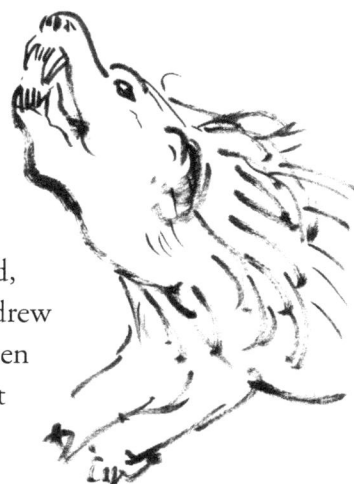

The patient will exhibit one of only three actions:

1. They keep on coming; you are now being assaulted. In this case you will do what you have to do to ensure safety.
2. They get *too* close and when you tell them to step back, they say, "Make me." Once again, this is an assault. You will do what you have to do to ensure safety.
3. They comply. When patients in hot rage comply with the command to step back, they usually do so yelling and screaming: "You can't tell me what to do!" or simply yelling obscenities. You should continue the Ladder and expect compliance at each 'rung.'

Once you have them de-escalated, you must maintain control. Only after setting very strong limits would you shift into problem-solving, even with a mentally ill patient. Otherwise, they will assume that the best way to get a reward—your attention or help—is to abuse you.

Hot Rage Subtype #2: Bluff-Rage
Taking Control of Them Includes 'Face Saving'

These patients, like gorillas beating their chests, display aggression to keep you at a distance, or otherwise make an impression. They're like a wind blowing against a stone-wall rather than like the pent-up explosiveness of dynamite under a rock.

Nonetheless, their manifest behavior appears much the same as the patient displaying fury, hence the terrifying image of the enraged gorilla. At 20 yards, could you really tell the difference between a charging gorilla and a charging grizzly bear? Both are huge, hairy beasts that apparently mean you harm. The gorilla, however, would prefer to be left alone, rather than engaging in combat. But he postures as if he wants nothing more than to tear you to pieces. And if he perceives no other alternative, he will.

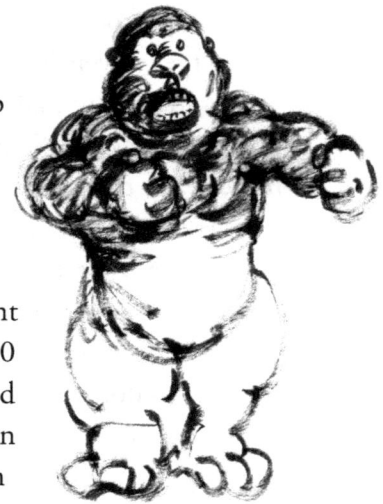

Those showing bluff-rage are often displaying aggression for the benefit of friends or family. *They're frightened that they will be found out as frightened.* They may be trying to impress others or convince them that they're someone to take seriously. Their friends or family members have, on many occasions, provoked them to 'prove' they are tough.

Figure 51.5 Difference Between a Furious Aggressor and a Bluffer

How do you know the difference between a furious aggressor and a bluffer, if their behavior is so close? When you are facing a furious person, fear is your natural and likely response. Your animal mind—that part of you that puts survival above all else—demands your attention now, and it uses fear to accomplish this. A bluffer, in a state of hot rage, will also elicit fear, but this will be accompanied by another emotion—irritation. You will be, to use the vernacular, 'pissed off,' thinking how stupid this incident has become, and that if the bluffer hadn't chosen to bring his friends, or if his wife hadn't chosen to taunt him as being less than a man, this dangerous situation would never have developed.

Warning: you still must take bluff-rage very seriously! If they do succeed in working themselves up, they will become violent. Such people can be quite dangerous for another reason. Because they're performing in front of an audience and afraid that those watching will realize that they're afraid, they will often attack if they feel found out for what they are. Many bullies, who have a long record of appalling violence, actually function in bluff mode. They're in a perpetual quest to prove to others—and even more insidiously, to themselves—that they aren't frightened. They repetitively solicit situations where they must either intimidate or beat someone bloody. Therefore, it is essential to short-circuit this behavior before it escalates into violence.

Sometimes bluffers are alone, but they still have an audience—the one inside their own head. They have an image inside their own mind to which they believe they must conform.

When the bluffer is frightened, he moves forward, not back, so that no one will see how scared he is.

Figure 51.6 Concerning a patient in Bluff-rage

It isn't helpful to empathize with them that you understand that they're scared underneath. You must take them seriously, just like you would a very big, threatening gorilla.

Control of Bluff-Rage

These patients aren't really in confrontation with you. They're *pretending* that they are. But this is a pretense that can kill. Use the Ladder, the same verbal control tactic you use with an enraged patient. Your tone, however, should be much more matter-of-fact and relaxed. Your eye-contact, too, is matter-of-fact, as if you're having a conversation rather than a confrontation. Rather than having your hands in front of you (clasped or in a 'fence'), open your hands, slightly to the sides, palm up. You're definitely prepared and able to protect yourself, if you need to, but at the same time, you aren't trying to frighten or intimidate them. You're, in essence, saying, "There is no fight here. But I'm so confident and in control that I certainly could handle myself if there was." Remember, they will attack out of fear. Your task is, paradoxically, to help them save face so that they willingly step-back rather than *forcing* them to do so.

Figure 51.7 The Bluffer's strut

When you have done things well, they often strut back with a smirk, sometimes glancing around and making eye-contact with their audience; this is for the benefit of the audience, and their own self-image. They're trying to show that they aren't afraid, and in control of the situation. Do NOT call them on this—they are saving face as they comply with what you want them to do.

In some situations, you can short circuit things before they become too intense by helping them save face. Include in your strategy some information and re-assurance. For example, you can say, "Look, Frank. I know you thought I was making fun of you, but that wasn't the case at all. I was just pointing out that you forgot your meds, so you wouldn't have to come back for them later." <u>Be careful that in doing so, you don't make the bluffer out to be a winner! Helping them save face must not mean that you have 'backed down' in a way that compromises your authority.</u> Furthermore, if they have ramped themselves into true 'bluff-rage,' they may view conceding a point with you as giving up. In these cases, only by taking total control will you be able to ensure your own and other's safety.

- Don't point out their fears in front of others. They will feel the need to defend their honor.

- If they aren't responsive to a more low-key approach and continue to escalate, you may have a furious aggressor who *happens* to be in front of other people or a bluffer who has shifted into fury. In this case, you 'turn up the dial,' and drop your voice to be low and powerful, shift into the ladder technique for the furious patient. In essence, you would say, "Move back, Stephen. We will talk about it——<then putting much more power in your words> MOVE BACK!, etc."

Just as with the furious aggressor, you must set limits at the end of the confrontation. However, you should also include some 'ego building.' These patients are most dangerous when they're depending on others to feel strong. Therefore, draw them aside, and say something like what is stated in the figure below:

Figure 51.8 Example of Communicating With a Person Under Control After Being in a Bluff-rage

"Bernard, I'm glad this worked out with no one getting hurt. Had you not chosen to sit down and talk, you very likely would have ended up hooked up by the cops over there. No. Listen to me for a minute. I'm not disrespecting you—that's why you and I are over here talking instead of in front of them <indicating the onlookers>. I'm telling you, it was a very near thing. Again, I'm glad this has worked out that you and I are standing here talking."

"Next time, though, don't do this in front of them" (referring to his friends or family for whom he was on display, and actually put a little *contempt* in your voice when you say the word 'them' as if to indicate that Bernard is better/cooler/stronger than those people he is trying to impress.)

"Come to me and talk to me one man to another" OR "one woman to another" ("one adult to another" in male-female conversations). "You shouldn't put your personal business in front of them." You will observe him 'puff up,' feeling flattered. You then continue, "Okay. Are we clear for next time? Good. Now as for this time…." Then set the same types of limits as you did with the patient in a state of FURY.

Remember, it is the audience that makes this patient most dangerous. If they feel that they will get 'respect' by themselves, if they believe their status will improve if they come in alone rather than with their crew of friends or family, they will be far less dangerous next time. This technique is advised when dealing with gangs. Face-saving is extremely important—a gang-affiliated individual is far less likely to impede you in your task when he or she is not performing in front of his/her associates. Though we don't care about them respecting us, they, paradoxically, care more about such respect, even from us, than they care for their lives or their friends.

Hot Rage Subtype #3: Aggressive-Manipulation
Taking Control Means Not 'Buying In' to the Game

Aggressive-manipulation is a *strategy*, not a symptom of illness. People displaying this type of behavior can have any one of a number of mental illnesses. Aggressive-manipulators are calculating, trying to monitor the effect of what they're doing. They don't care about honor, integrity, or pride. All they want to do is win any way they can. You can sometimes tell when you're being manipulated ('played') because you're confused about why the person is upset, or what is the purpose of the argument. The aggressive-manipulator frequently changes either his/her mood or the subject of the complaint.

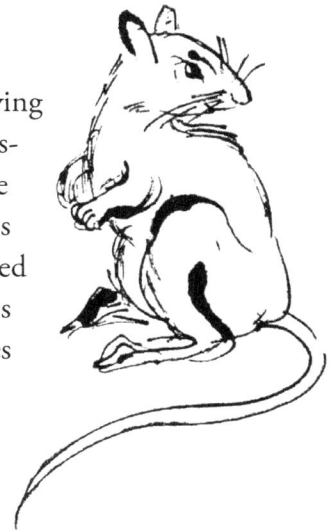

Aggressive manipulative people may have a long history of losing control, particularly when their desires are frustrated, or when they believe they aren't given what they believe they're entitled to. Very frequently they have a history of personality disorder (particularly with sociopathic, anti-social, paranoid, narcissistic, borderline or histrionic character traits).

The opportunistic-manipulative individual will show a number of strategies to facility aggression:

- They might start with a plea for something, talking about how they're suffering, but once refused, they blame or criticize you.
- They may try to seduce you, "C'mon, I just smacked my kid. That's not abuse. You aren't going to call the cops for just disciplining my kid? C'mon, you know me!"
- They might try to make you feel guilty and then start demeaning you verbally, if you do not respond. This may shift to allusions or threats of violence.
- They may talk in an arrogant manner, trying to make you look incompetent or stupid.
- They often claim to be a victim, basing this on either real or imaginary issues. Furthermore, they may use their 'status' as a member of an oppressed or victimized class of people as a means of intimidating others or making them feel off-balance.
- They may make their demands in a whiny, accusatory voice. They will footnote old grievances, bringing up trivia, accusations and old history. They will tell you how you're just like someone else who "did them wrong."
- They ask frequent and repetitive questions, and try to frighten you or make you feel uncertain of yourself.

We often use the image of a large rat, because rats are the ultimate survivors. They will do whatever it takes to win. This image is not intended to be demeaning. It merely underscores that aggressive-manipulators, like our furry, long-tailed cousins, are infinitely adaptable and whatever the conditions, will attempt to find a way to endure or win.

Manipulation doesn't mean false threat. Manipulative people will often harm others—some will even kill. The difference between such an aggressive-manipulator and those in a state of pure fury is that the furious are swept by their rage. We say, "He lost it." The aggressive-manipulator attempts to monitor your responses and the situation *while aggressing* to assess if what he/she is doing is the best way to get what they want. The opportunistic/manipulator is, therefore, calculating. However, that doesn't mean that he/she is in control. As they gets more and more agitated, their judgment deteriorates, and they may concoct a rationalization for violence that makes sense to them in the moment—even when it would to no one else

The idea of 'intimidation for next time,' as stupid as it sounds, is the driver of some aggressive-manipulators. Imagine a large male facing a young 5 foot 3 inch female EMT. Such a patient thinks that he will be able to put some significant damage on this person before subdued. As far as he is concerned, the damage he will inflict is worth the damage he might receive, because he thinks that the 'history' he is making will cause people to treat him differently next time.

Control Tactics for Aggressive-manipulators

People who use this strategy of attack are, by definition, acting in a degraded manner because they're trying to twist your feelings (making you feel guilty, ashamed, off-balance, or scared), or trying to trick you to get what they want. Don't buy in to it: <u>If you catch them using this strategy early, cut it off at the onset. Verbally suppress any and all verbal gambits.</u>

If however, the manipulative-aggressor begins to escalate his/her strategies, you may have to use the Ladder as you put them under control. With these people, you can and should use the Ladder *even before* they shift into rage—view their manipulative verbal games as the first initiation of their attack.

At the early stages (when things are purely verbal), look past one ear rather than making eye contact. Making eye contact allows them to get information from you. Aggressive-manipulative people don't care about you—they use eye contact to 'read' you and control you. They're interested in what they can use when you reveal yourself to them. Similarly, they will use their own eyes to create a false intimacy—they 'reveal' both truth *and* falsehood to confuse you, misdirect your attention, or dominate you. Your disinterested look conveys, "I'm not in your game," and also shows a kind of strong dominance—indicating you won't lower yourself to their currently degraded level. Such disinterest is also revealed in your vocal tone, which should be matter-of fact and slightly detached.

Figure 51.9 Don't Look Away

Don't look away. While looking past an ear, you can still see what they're doing. If you look away, you will be assaulted and not even know it is coming. This disengaged look, done properly, indicates that you won't participate in the degradation that manipulation creates.

Aggressive-manipulative rage is distinguished from pure fury in that, even now, they're attempting to read and monitor you for advantage: are they intimidating you; have they succeeded in distracting or throwing you off balance so that you're open to an attack; have they got you trying to "bargain" your way to safety? At the same time, they will begin to 'lose it,' as their strategic application of intimidation is unsuccessful. They get frustrated because they believe their manipulation *should* be working. In essence, aggressive-manipulative rage is a merger of hot rage (fury) and predatory rage (Chapters 51 and 52).

- Stand relaxed and ready to evade a blow and counter the attack.
- Express flat disinterest in their demands, accusations, and complaints.
- Use the repetitive commands of the Ladder technique. Your vocal tone is flat. Don't negotiate. Don't discuss anything as long as they're using this kind of degraded behavior.

With the aggressive-manipulative patient, several things can happen when you attempt to control their escalation:

- Your flat disinterest means to them that they can't 'get to you.' After trying several different avenues, they shift to another strategy, or give up in defeat.
- In more heated situations, they will flare into a fury or pseudo-fury (the latter for the purpose of intimidation). At this point, lock eyes with a small head roll, a 'loop,' very similar to what you do with your teenage child (or your parents did with you), and inform them that they must stop the behavior..
- When you 'lock in' eye-contact, they may 'bounce' off into another tactic—sudden tears, for example.

If they flare into pure fury, manage their behavior just like any other patient in a state of fury.

Figure 51.10 Important: Locking Eyes—The Loop

If they flare into *fury* or if they continue to be non-compliant, turn from looking past the ear to looking right in their eyes with a firm command to stop what they're doing. When you turn you head to look directly in their eyes, roll it slightly up and then down as if sighting a weapon. Speak powerfully and directly, just as you do with the patient who is in a state of fury. If they don't stop immediately upon being 'hit' with your eyes, this means that an attack is imminent. You will shift into the de-escalation for fury or even further, take action to ensure your safety in the event of violence.

CHAPTER 52

Predatory Or Cool Rage

Thankfully, this type of individual is rather rare. Such people are like a panther or a shark. (The distinction is that the 'panther' can be charming or personally attractive, whereas the 'shark' is just a dangerous being, whose potential for violence is unambiguously clear). They're intimidators who threaten either with vague innuendoes or explicit threats. Their behavior is calculated, but unlike the aggressive-manipulator, violence is often their first choice rather than one of many options. The predator delivers threats in cool, dangerous tones, often *after* a clear and strongly stated demand. Then they offer you a chance *not to be injured* if you comply with their demand. A variant tactic is to pretend being out of control. (This is in contrast to a genuine attack, an action that they're eminently capable, and willing, to carry out).

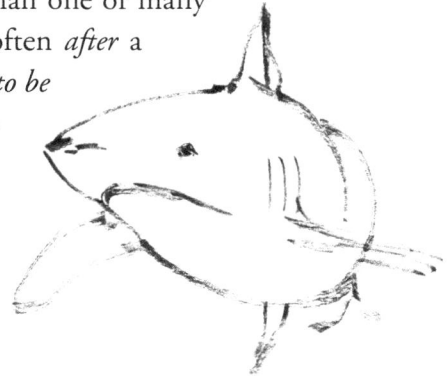

These individuals seethe with hostility and/or contempt for other people, but they have developed the application of these emotions as a deliberate weapon of terror or even enjoyment. Paradoxically, many experience low levels of anxiety in situations that would frighten ordinary people. Their heart rate can actually go down as they prepare to commit violence. They can be charming and attractive, as fictional pirates are when not being aggressive. Therefore, some people may have a hard time believing that they're so capable of terrorizing others psychologically, or hurting them physically, because they can act like such nice people. These people, either situationally (the 'professional' criminal) or pervasively (the sociopath) lack a moral sensibility or conscience. Nothing inhibits their aggression other than tactical calculation or self-interest: they have no capacity for sympathy or guilt. Every time they intimidate someone, their behavior is reinforced. They take non-action on your part as either the behavior of weak prey or of tacit approval of what they do.

The best response is a combination of overwhelming force and respect.[32] The former is obvious. Strive to never be in a situation where you're vulnerable with such a patient. 'Respect' means, simply, that you make your control 'institutional,' not 'personal.'

There are, however, times, where you have gotten over the 'horizon line,' and you do not have either back-up or a suitable escape route. Imagine, for example, being accosted at a shopping center, with your children, whom you don't want to expose to the predator. He/she hasn't seen your kids yet, and you don't want them to.

Your basic task is to demonstrate that you aren't prey, that it would take too much effort on the predator's part to hurt you. It may be that you create an impression that you're another predator. That isn't necessary, however. It is enough that he/she sees you as not 'edible,' like an animal with quills or one that would taste bad:

- Stand ready to move. Be poised, but not too defensive.
- Be open and strategic in everything you do—the way you position your body, your voice, and your posture. He/she is a professional at reading weakness, at delving out what you're trying to hide. Therefore, protect yourself openly. If he/she says something like, "You think stepping back is going to help you?" ignore it and act in your best interests. Don't change your actions based on what he/she says.
- He/she will try to use anything you do against you, either deriding you or pretending that you're out of control, paranoid, or acting strangely. Ignore all that and act to keep yourself safe.

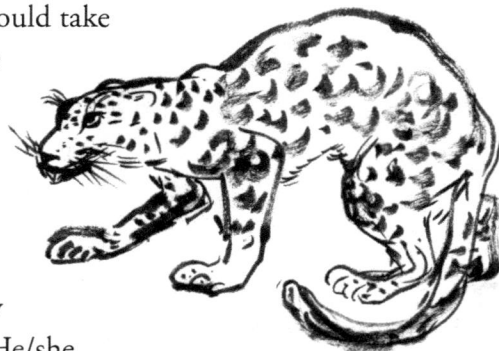

Cryptic Consequences: Your Strategic Response to the Predator

Keep your voice matter-of-fact, and give clear and direct statements of *potential* consequences. If you can, smile. <u>These consequences are of a special type, clear, but cryptic,</u> e.g., "You know what would happen if you did that." In this case, don't tell them what would happen. Let their imagination take over. These vague consequences are a mirror of their own method of intimidation, and they may react to you as 'not prey, not edible, not worth the trouble.'

- If they say, "What are you talking about?" you should reply, "You know exactly what I are talking about." When the predator responds to your cryptic consequence with questions or with confusing statements that would make your statement illogical, simply say, "You know what is going on here. You know what is happening."
- You may have to intersperse your vague consequences with Ladder commands if they escalate their behavior.
- Don't get 'caught' in their eyes. However, you need to look directly at them, so look between their eyes, or look with an empty stare (imagine turning your eyes to buttons. He/she will look like a cut-out or silhouette). Your eyes are flat, with no attempt to 'penetrate' or make contact. (You should make sustained eye-contact only if in a fight for your life. Then, you must shift focus, trying to penetrate his/her eyes as if you were a laser beam).
- Don't over-react to threats, or they will interpret your reaction as a victory.
- Your entire goal is to convince them that it isn't worth it to hurt you. Once you have succeeded and are free, you need to get help.

To reiterate, you don't have to prove that you're bigger, tougher, or more dangerous. You're establishing that you're merely on to their game and aren't, by nature, someone to victimize. Like a leopard who chooses *not* to chase an antelope because it is moving too smoothly, showing that it is healthy and strong, the predator is likely to disengage if you don't give him anything to brush off (an attempt to intimidate them with a direct threat) or if you try to negotiate (something they have no interest in).

Figure 52.1 An Explicit Threat Is an Empty Threat

Particularly when you don't have the overwhelming force component **don't** make explicit threats, such as "If you come near my family, I will kill you!" That tells them what you *won't* do. In their mind, if you really meant it, you would do it now. They think, "I'm serious. I mean what I'm going to do. He/she knows it, but all they can do is tell me what they're going to do after I do what I'm going to do." An explicit threat is an empty threat.

Figure 52.2 Example of a cryptic interaction with predatory patient.

"Look, this is very simple. I think you and I can agree that you misinterpreted what I said about hitting my wife. I don't know where you got the idea that I said I beat her. Look, I understand. You must have been having a bad day, and you over-reacted. This can be fixed very easily. Just call the cops and tell them that you didn't quote me accurately, that you've been overworked lately and misjudged the situation. See, I bet you love your family as much as I do. You've got your child in a good school over at Echo Lake. Actually, it's amazing, that's one of the last schools in this area that still lets the kids out for recess. It's nice to see little kids playing so happily and innocently.

Oh, sorry, I'm a little off track. What I'm saying is that I bet you would be devastated if anything happened to your family. I'm the same. The problem here is that what is happening to my family is you! And this is a problem you could fix, unless you are really sitting there telling me that you want to destroy my life and that of my child. IS THAT WHAT YOU ARE SAYING??!!!!"

You. *(With a little smile and a strong, confident voice)* "I'm really glad we're having this conversation, because it's good that we both understand each other."

Predator. "So you'll make the call."

You. "Oh, you know what's going to happen."

Predator. "Suppose you tell me."

You. "There's no need to do that. You know exactly what's going on."

Predator. *(Getting a little confused)* "Are you threatening me?"

You. "I don't know where you got that idea. In fact, we both know the situation here."

Predator. *(Walking away after a hard stare)* "You think this is over. You better watch your back."

Please note that this exchange could conceivably go on for a longer period of time. We are here presenting enough back-and-forth that you should clearly understand the principle.

As soon as you have achieved your goal of separating yourself from the predator, call law enforcement. As you and your family have been threatened (whether the tone is velvet or harsh), you must do everything necessary to keep everyone safe. You may have to be on your guard for a long time. Such incidents are sometimes just words, or sometimes just a one-time affair, but on other occasions, they can go on for a long time, with further threats, stalking or other dangerous behaviors that require you to muster all professional skills and assistance to ensure that you and your family are safe.

Figure 52.3 CAUTION

You ONLY use this strategy with the openly predatory, that most rare of people, and ONLY when they're escalating into predatory rage, <u>and only when you don't have sufficient force or backup.</u> In other words, it should never happen, but you need to know what to do if it does.

CHAPTER 53

Deceptive Rage:
Snake In The Grass

Many criminals have concurrent mental illnesses; others have spent time in a forensic unit somewhere for evaluation purposes; still others are there because they were able to fake mental illness so that they could be moved to a hospital either for a more attractive environment, or for the purposes of escape.

What do you think such individuals do, particularly the manipulative and sociopathic, while in the hospital? They victimize more vulnerable patients, either directly, or indirectly. Their opportunities to torment the genuinely mentally ill are endless.

Beyond such predation, they study, because who knows, perhaps the behaviors of a mentally ill individual may prove advantageous someday. Perhaps it will prove useful in convincing an evaluator that they are genuinely mentally ill and of diminished capacity, not responsible for the crime they committed. Furthermore, perhaps it will give such a person an opportunity to catch someone off guard, even a firefighter or EMT.

Such an individual obscures his/her intentions behind a screen behavior: the imitation of genuinely mentally ill individuals whom they have observed. They pretend to be psychotic, in a state of terror, distressed or needing your help. All this is for the purpose of either conning you into leaving them alone, or more dangerously, drawing you close enough so they can harm you.

Imagine a snake coiled in the leaves, pattern almost indiscernible from the ground, ready to strike.

The 'de-escalation' strategy here is simple: deal with the behavior, not the cause! Imagine you are attempting to treat a confused, psychotic-appearing patient. You have police back-up. They do not realize that this individual is actually a subject of interest in a crime in another jurisdiction. What you don't realize is that before you arrived, he was absolutely cognitively intact. When you arrived with police, lolling his head, thrusting his tongue out and answering your questions in tangential, apparently confused fashion. He tells you that he was just released from a crisis unit in another state and doesn't have identification. His eyes are a little teary, and he looks so intimidated and

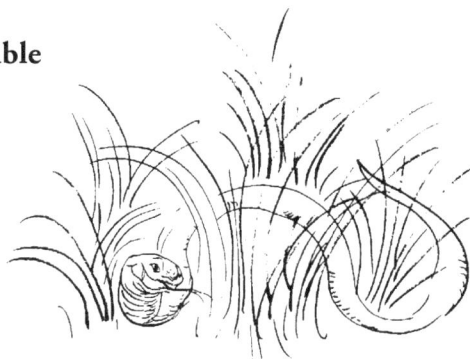

he hunches over a little as he cries, but <u>you can't see his hands</u>! You ask to see his hands and he thrusts one deeper in his pocket. What should you do?

1. In this case, you step back, point out to the police officer that the patient is hiding his hands, and request that the officer take control to assure safety.

2. If this incident occurred without police presence, get some distance between you, and you order them to show you their hands. If they do not immediately comply, remove yourself and your crew from the scene.

In general, one of two things will result:

- A predatory individual, they slowly remove their hand and exercising due caution, a police officer pats them down and find a shank (or you have removed yourself from the presence of an individual who, if you got closer, might have stabbed you).

- They are genuinely mentally ill or developmentally disabled, and at your sharp command, they begin crying in terror. You are now in the position of helping them. Once you ascertain everything is safe, you kindly but firmly tell them that you are going to teach them the rules of how to talk with first responders. "I'm sorry you were frightened. But you did something that looked dangerous. I'll tell you right now how you should act so something like this won't happen again."

CHAPTER 54

Feeding Frenzy—
Mob Rage

Figure 54.1 Rage State and Possibility of Violence

This discussion covers both the rage state and the possibility of violence. Pack behavior can easily escalate and therefore, it is impossible to separate rage from violence in this discussion. The discussion here concerns situations where you don't have sufficient forces to manage the mob.

Pack behavior amplifies hot rage exponentially—one person's arousal ramping up those around. The more people there are, the more likely that one will create an enraged mob, a beast of many heads, but one terrifying, destructive mind. People in the mob will manifest any one of the types of rage, including terrified, chaotic, fury, bluff, manipulation and predatory. Sometimes mob frenzy is created and stoked by one predator, who coolly uses the mob as a weapon.

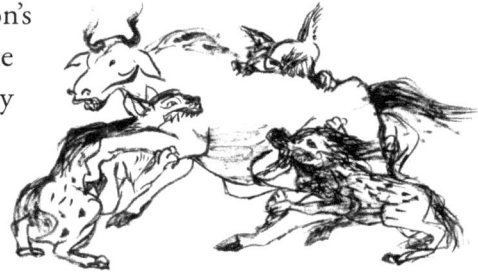

The sum total is frenzy. If you're caught in such a group, GET OUT QUICKLY. Within a mass, people lose any sense of compassion or guilt and they believe there is anonymity within the mass. Note the grinning faces of people in photos of lynch mobs—all the inhibitors against violation of another melt away within the ecstasy of the group mind.

Intervention with a Group or a Mob

Horribly, you might be in a situation where you shouldn't or can't escape— because there is no escape route, because you're responsible for the safety of others, or if the mob is just coalescing—if you step in now, you may be able to diffuse things:

- **Overwhelming force.** Quite simply, the most powerful method of de-escalation is a demonstration to the mob and its members that they will be stopped. Each member of the mob suddenly feels alone—"the first to go down."
- **Isolate the leader.** Isolating the leader as the one person who will face the consequences. All of your psychological energy should be focused on the leader. This is particularly powerful when the leader is hiding behind the power of the mob. If you perceive that the leader is manifesting manipulative, bluff, or predatory rage, make it clear that whatever happens, they won't emerge unscathed. The goal is definitely not to shame them. If you present yourself absolute calm, speak-

ing to him or her in a quiet matter-of-fact tone, the mob leader can save face. This is essential if you have any hope of causing him to draw his forces back.

- **Build up the leader's ego.** When it is clear that the leader is trying to puff up his/her ego through the mob, make it clear he or she is the only one worthy of conferring with you. This is for the purpose of either drawing them away from the group, so he/she can't wield them against you, or to appeal to their grandiose narcissism. If his/her goal is to appear important in the eyes of the mob, you may have given him/her what they really want, without the need for violence.
- **Break the pattern.** As discussed in Chapter 44, you do something so unexpected or outlandish that none of the patients in the mob knows how to react. A police officer from Belfast, Northern Ireland wrote to one of the authors that during what was possibly a build up to a riot, he played ice cream truck music from his cellular phone over the public address system in his vehicle. This resulted in the de-escalation of the situation but unfortunately "some senior police brass didn't approve and I was spoken to about my behavior."

To reiterate, the best option when facing a mob, whenever possible, is to tactically remove yourself and your crew to a safer position and summon assistance. If you do intervene, be aware that you may have to fight for your life. Your best hope, were this terrible situation to develop is 'to go berserk,' using any weapon you can get in your hands. Be like a wolverine in a trap with teeth, claws and anything else you can use, try to tear your way free. To put it directly, you are trying to maim your attackers as savagely as you can. The goal is to become so appallingly violent that each member of the group wants to get away from you. As they recoil, hopefully, an escape route may open up.

CHAPTER 55

The Aftermath—What Happens Internally To The Aggressive, Mentally Ill Patient After An Aggressive Incident?

Rage and even more so, violence, are exhausting experiences—both emotionally and physically. Many people get the 'shakes' after such an event. So much blood has 'pooled' inside the core of their bodies to prepare for combat that they feel cold and start to tremble. Most patients have a significantly impaired ability to remember what happened in sequence. They may have a patchy memory of a few events. Much of the rest of the incident is a blur. Although they may be remorseful, they usually don't remember what happened, how it started, or who was responsible. Even more drastically, they can lapse into a state of defensive confusion where they no longer recall what happened at all, or they distort the incident in their memory completely, thereafter taking no responsibility whatsoever.

Others may feel profound guilt. This might be positive, were it to lead them to reflect on their own responsibility, but for most people, this guilt is so noxious that they project responsibility onto the person who 'makes' them feel guilty. Thus, they soon shift to resentment and begin to blame the other person.

It is quite common that the patient experiences humiliation, the feeling of having one's faults or vulnerabilities exposed to others, and here, too, many people become defensive. People describe humiliation like being flayed and exposed. Some respond to shame by becoming enraged all over again. Their thinking seems to be, "If I feel this bad, someone must be doing it to me." What is almost universal is a post–crisis fatigue, a combination of the depletion of energy stores in the body and the cumulative effect of all the mood and cognitive changes described above.

Managing Risks Post-Crisis

You may have to 'take care' of the patient, particularly if they're mentally ill or developmentally disabled. Even if you have successfully controlled them so that they didn't commit an act of violence, you still may have a role in helping keep them stable while they are being seen at a hospital, crisis triage center, or even in the field. Your tasks may include maintaining control, and establish limits and consequences. You may even need to possibly regain rapport and provide reassurance.

If the patient is someone who can accept feedback and help after the crisis is resolved, your first responsibility is clarification—clearly delineating what was abusive, aggressive, or otherwise unacceptable behavior.

If a patient, perhaps severely mentally ill, is really frightened, or devastated by what happened, the first priority is <u>reassurance and orientation</u>—letting them know that they aren't going to be punished (this, of course, is different from consequences—in other words, no one is going to take revenge on them, something the more paranoid will expect). In cases with people who are demented, psychotic, or otherwise in fragile mental states, you may have to explain to them what has happened, where they are, what is going to happen now, and who you are, etc. If patients do have cognitive abilities and are calm enough to understand, <u>educative follow-up</u> should include:

- Discussing what other tactics they might have used to get what they desired;
- Assisting them in becoming aware of patterns that led up to the aggression or assault;
- Negotiating agreements on how to avoid such incidents in the future;
- Assisting the patient to return to a sense of dignity and integrity.

Some people aren't suited to have such a debriefing. Developmentally disabled patients, or others with dementia or cognitive impairments can't really remember what happened, and they may re-escalate thinking they're, once again, under attack. With people who don't have the mental capacity to really understand the details or implications of what happened, it is better to be calming and reassuring, not problem-solving.

CHAPTER 56

Conclusion

As you have read, this is far more than just 'how to deal with patients with mentally illness.' We deal with all kinds of people, of any age, shape, or size. Anyone can be dangerous—and we must have a 'best practice' response to each.

It is important that you regularly review and practice the safety and de-escalation methods in this book. You should be as familiar with this information as you are with the skills necessary to start an intravenous line, intubate a patient, administer medications or perform other medical procedures. Just as you automatically snatch your hand away from a hot stove or blink your eyes when a small object flies toward them, these skills must become so familiar to you that they seem as reflexive as instincts.

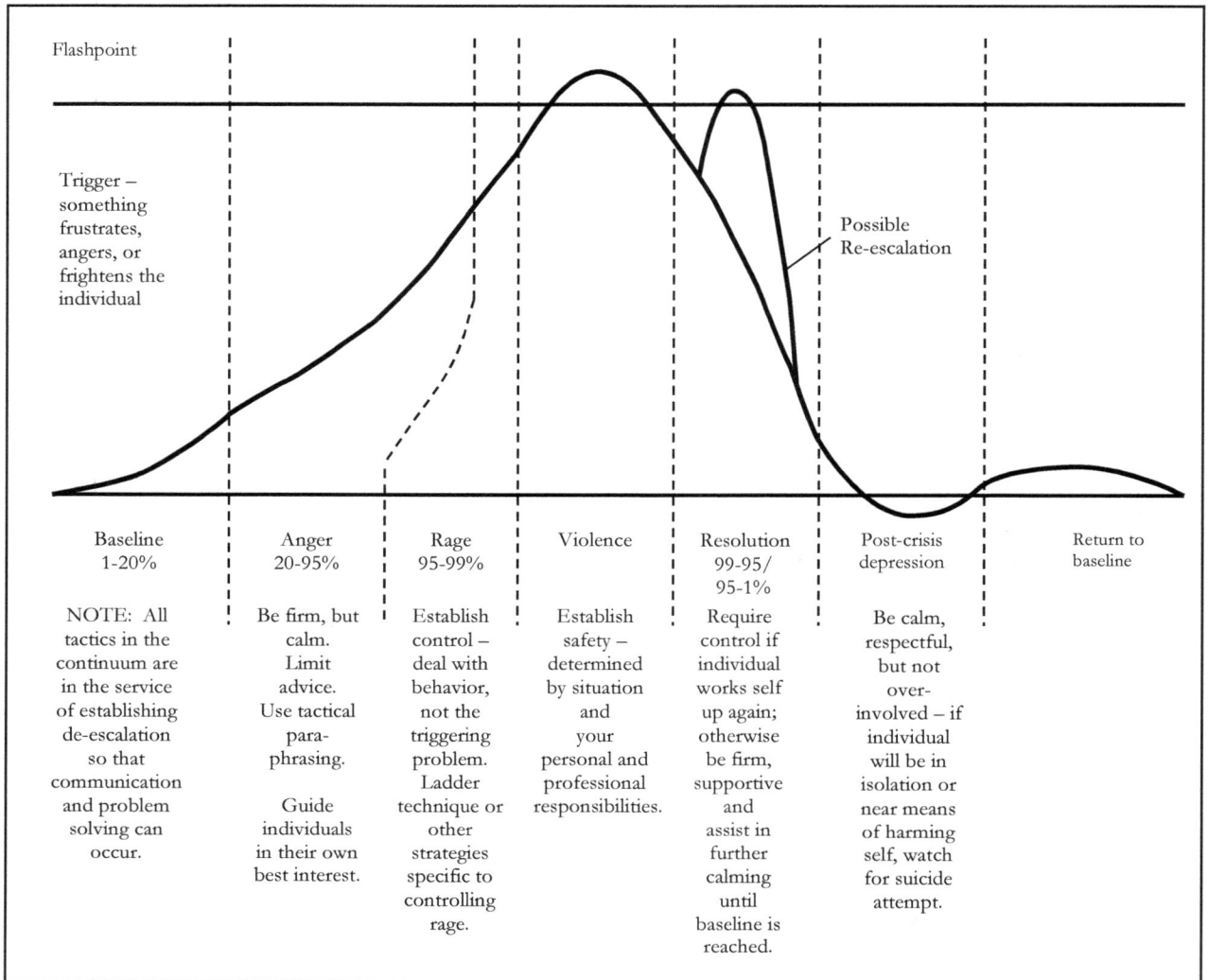

Flashpoint

Trigger –
something
frustrates,
angers, or
frightens the
individual

Possible
Re-escalation

Baseline 1-20%	Anger 20-95%	Rage 95-99%	Violence	Resolution 99-95/ 95-1%	Post-crisis depression	Return to baseline
NOTE: All tactics in the continuum are in the service of establishing de-escalation so that communication and problem solving can occur.	Be firm, but calm. Limit advice. Use tactical para-phrasing. Guide individuals in their own best interest.	Establish control – deal with behavior, not the triggering problem. Ladder technique or other strategies specific to controlling rage.	Establish safety – determined by situation and your personal and professional responsibilities.	Require control if individual works self up again; otherwise be firm, supportive and assist in further calming until baseline is reached.	Be calm, respectful, but not over-involved – if individual will be in isolation or near means of harming self, watch for suicide attempt.	

Appendices

APPENDIX A

Physical And Chemical Restraint
Of Patients

Use of Restraints

Restraining your patients is a process that needs to be well thought out. Events that require restraint of patients often occur suddenly, and your crew cannot invent procedures in the middle of an emergency, particularly when you are attacked or assaulted. Therefore, policies and procedures need to be established well before the event occurs.

Any restraint procedure must be outlined within your department's EMS protocols. First responders MUST train and frequently practice effective restraint procedures, thereby minimizing the risk of injury or even death to your patient. Beyond this, it is imperative that firefighters and EMT cross-train with law enforcement personnel:

- One of the most dangerous points in situations requiring restraint is the transition from police control to medical restraint. If this is not well-coordinated, patients as well as first responders can be injured.
- Chemical restraints are sometimes administered while the patient is under the control of law enforcement. In cases of chaotic rage (Chapter 49 & Appendix C), this can be while the person is still undergoing the effects of an electronic control device (TASER™). Firefighters, paramedics and EMTs must know how best to coordinate their actions with law enforcement to effectively administer chemical restraint in these circumstances, and in particular, not get 'tazed' themselves by getting tangled up in the wires.

There are two major categories of restraint: physical restraints, which start with a take-down and hold-down through to the use of devices such as straps, belts, webbing or some other form of soft restraints, and chemical restraints with the use of medications.

There is not one ironclad standard of practice concerning restraint procedures. However, standards of practice should conform to current research-based information, not anecdote or outdated, unsubstantiated procedures. Acceptable procedures are mediated by state law, local ordinances, and are often derived from protocols of mental health agencies or hospitals. (See Appendix B on the current state of knowledge and research concerning so-called 'positional asphyxiation' and 'restraint asphyxiation.')

There is a consensus, reflected in most guidelines that encourages the judicious use of restraints: using minimal force to restrain a patient; ensuring there is a police presence, whenever possible, when dealing with a potentially or actually combative patient,; and communication with your medical control point before restraining a patient whenever possible.

There are all too many examples of improper restraint, including the use of excessive force, or positioning in such a way that the patient's breathing is compromised. A best practice is to use the least restrictive alternative to protect a patient from harming or others. If wrist restraints and gentle pressure on the hips, legs and shoulders accomplishes the task, then use that method. If unsuccessful, the first responder must use greater restraint methodology to control the patient. If there is an immediate danger to the patient or first responders, overwhelming force by the attendant first responders to subdue or control the patient may be required.

Chemical restraints, either in coordination or in lieu of physical restraint, involve the use of medication. The usual medication types are antipsychotics, benzodiazepines, and increasingly, Ketamine, as they are less invasive and cause less injury to the patient or first responder.

In many, if not most EMS systems, the protocols addressing the use of restraining devices, in many circumstances require the EMTs or paramedics to call Medical Control first to obtain permission to restrain a patient or to involve the local police in the restraining procedures.

Not all restraining requires prior medical control approval:
- It is not unlawful to 'strap and load' patients, if that is accepted professional practice and the action is taken in the patient's best interests (not the paramedic's convenience) and the patient consents (either expressly or by implication e.g. by cooperating with the process);
- It is not unlawful to restrain a person if that is accepted professional practice and the action is taken in the patient's best interests (not the paramedic or EMTs convenience) and, if the patient is unable to consent, the decision is reasonable in the circumstances and in the patient's best interests;
- It is not unlawful to restrain a person who is suffering a mental illness if that is accepted professional practice (which may require seeking some endorsement from the medical director if that is the procedure adopted in the approved protocols), and the paramedic believes, based on reasonable grounds, that such action is necessary to protect the patient or other people who may be at risk (such as paramedics or a police officer in the ambulance).

The use of chemical restraints must be in accordance with training, and the paramedics or qualified EMTs must use drugs that are authorized for that purpose.

Appendix A: Figure 1 – Police do not make the decision for medical restraint.

The mere request made by a police officer for the firefighter, paramedics or EMTs to restrain the patient is not sufficient. If they are transporting the person, it is their professional duty to act in their patient's best interests and that may well mean resisting a police officer's desire to unnecessarily restrain the patient. It's not for police to tell paramedics how to apply a restraint any more than a police officer will direct a paramedic how to treat a person with a traumatic injury.

Comprehensive training and frequent practice is required to be effective at restraint procedures. Complete protocols must include:

1. A definition of the reason and purpose of restraint
2. Attempts to use non-physical means of intervention, whenever possible, depending on the level of aggression (the subject of this book)
3. Types of physical restraints to be used
   a. Physical force—requiring adequate, well-trained personnel
   b. Strapping or belting systems, including acceptable types
4. Use of medications – Chemical Restraints
   a. Types and doses
5. Release protocols (this includes the transition from firefighter/EMT control to that of the hospital, jail or police), including:
   a. Hospital staff
   b. Police
   c. Jail
6. Transport times
   a. Short
   b. Long
7. Transportation Modalities and when each should be used.
   a. Ground
   b. Air

Example of a Training Directive

All paramedics and EMTs having direct contact with those patients who may cause harm to themselves or others must have ongoing education, training and demonstrated knowledge, on a regular basis, of:

1. Techniques to identify behaviors, events, and environmental factors that trigger emergency safety situations;
2. The use of nonphysical interventions skills, such as de-escalation, mediation, conflict resolution, tactical paraphrasing, verbal control tactics specific to different modes of rage, and verbal and observational methods, to prevent emergency safety situations;

3. The safe use of restraint (physical and/or chemical), including the ability to recognize and respond to signs of physical distress in individuals who are restrained or in seclusion.

Patients have the right to refuse treatment and/or transport if they are of legal age, and are determined by the first responder to be competent. Competence is defined as the capacity or ability to understand the nature and effects of one's acts or decisions. A person is considered to be competent until proven otherwise. There are situations, however, where the interests of the general public outweigh an individual's right to liberty:

1. The individual is threatening self-harm or suicide.
2. The individual presents a threat to the community because of a contagious disease or other physical dangerousness.
3. The individual presents a specific threat to innocent third parties.

Certain medical, traumatic and psychological conditions can cause incompetence and behavior that interferes with the ability of EMS personnel to care for the patient, or that threatens the physical wellbeing and safety of the patient or others. These conditions include, but are not limited to: drugs, metabolic disturbances, central nervous system injury or insult, infections, hypo/hypertension, hypo/hyperthermia, hypoxia, psychological disorders, poisons and toxins.

Example of State Regulation Concerning Physical Restraint

An example of a state regulation can be found in Washington State law,[33] that authorizes the use of reasonable force upon or toward the person without the other's consent when the following circumstances exist or the actor reasonably believes them to exist (Every state has similar statutes, and this is included as a typical example, not a proscription):

- When used to restrain a mentally ill or mentally impaired person from self injury or injury to another
- When used by one with authority to do so to compel compliance with reasonable requirements for the person's control, conduct or treatment.

This authority is found in RCW 9A.16.020 Use of force—When lawful, Section (6), and is used by any person to prevent a mentally ill, mentally incompetent, or mentally disabled person from committing an act dangerous to any person, or in enforcing necessary restraint for the protection or restoration to health of the person, during such period only as is necessary to obtain legal authority for the restraint or custody of the person.

If a first responder feels uncomfortable with any patient, even when they have not been actively combative, the provider has the right and duty to provide the patient and others with the security of patient restraint. Verbal threats are a legitimate reason for restraint.

Suggested Guidelines for Restraining a Patient in a Pre-Hospital Setting

1. Do everything possible to calm rather than aggravate an already tense situation.
2. Use de-escalation techniques (such as outlined in this book), to calm a patient.
3. Use the least restrictive means of control
4. Use reasonable force
5. Restraint may be required when you observe:
   - Patient behavior or threat creating a danger to the patient or others
   - A deterioration of a patient's condition which puts them or others at risk
   - An incompetent or combative patient.
6. Make sure you have adequate trained personnel if you are forcing a restraint—at least one per limb
7. Search the patient for any weapons (NOTE: it should go without saying that this should be a complete search—too many first responders have been injured, even killed, when they merely 'went through the motions' of a search.
8. For safety purposes, a restrained patient should be transported by ground ambulance and not via a helicopter.
9. The first responder must be constantly aware that medical equipment, as well as items in a car or home may be used a weapon. Therefore, ensuring scene safety is more than taking note of environmental hazards to the patient or crew—it includes the removal or securing of anything that a combative patient might use as a weapon.
10. Do not place patients in any position that may compromise breathing. If it is necessary to execute any restraint procedure *that has any possibility of compromising breathing*, check the patient every 3-5 minutes for patient airway and a pulse. Pregnant patients restrained must be placed on the left lateral recumbent position to not compromise fetal circulation. (See Appendix B for current [2015] information regarding research on 'positional asphyxiation' and 'restraint asphyxiation.')

For combative patients and when protocols allow, use the most appropriate medications to calm and sedate a patient.

Medical documentation of any restraint is imperative for medical records, and also to legally protect the first responder agency. If medical control was contacted prior to implementation of any restraining maneuver, ensure that the name of the authorizing physician is placed in the record. Make sure there is sequential documentation of the vital signs of the restrained patient.

A Sample Protocol Derived from Various Agencies[34]

Appendix A: Figure 2 – The conflict of best practices vs. established protocols

This section includes information that we consider as 'best practice,' derived from protocols from various agencies within the State of Washington for the use of physical and chemical restraints. We have included these in order that the reader can consider elements that can be integrated into your own protocols. These can be adopted, in part or in toto by EMS programs with the concurrence of the Medical Program Director, state law and after a review by the EMS program attorney or State's Attorney General Office.

Note Appendix B, concerning the most current research on the subject of positional asphyxia. Appendix C contains the Multiple Officer Control Tactic (MOCT) protocols, which we consider 'best practice' for physical restraint, as well as a detailed protocol on procedures to manage cases of chaotic rage/excited delirium.

We recommend that if readers wish to revamp their own restraint protocols, they should ensure due diligence regarding current procedures and best practices. Contact Edgework for if you wish to contact our subject-matter experts who developed Appendixes B & C.

Essential Aspects to a Protocol for Restraints

Prologue—Safety for EMS

Safety of the responding EMS providers has priority over patient care at all times. EMS personnel shall not enter into or remain in any situation that poses a threat to the safety of the team. Assuring the safety of the patient is then the second highest priority in treatment. Patients in hazardous or threatening environments should be protected or removed to a safe place before any definitive care is rendered. The EMS team members should enter the scene together, and generally, depart together. The assessment of scene safety is shared, but each individual EMS responder has the authority to decline to enter a potentially hazardous scene, or elect to leave. If any EMS team member is uncomfortable with the situation, and wants to leave, all team members should leave immediately.

Summon law enforcement at the first indication of danger

A patient is considered dangerous when the assessment indicates that the patient is:
- A threat to him/herself
- A threat to others
- Unable to care for him/herself and with potential underlying medical problems that are possibly masked by drugs, alcohol, mental illness, or head injury.

When a Patient is Not Aggressive or Combative

1. Approach the patient in a calm manner.
2. Show self-confidence and convey concern for the patient.
3. Reassure the patient he/she should and will be taken to a hospital where there are people who are interested in helping him/her.
4. One EMT should establish rapport and deal with the patient.

General Principles When Treating a Patient with Apparent Mental Illness or Emotional Disregulation

1. Transport the patient as quickly as possible without causing undo emotional or physical harm.
2. Contact police whenever a patient presents a risk of harm to self-or-others
3. If a medically-compromised patient, or one at risk of harm to self-or-others, appears to have a significant mental disorder and is refusing transport, it is best to involve police and/or mental health professional assistance, even if they are not combative.
4. Never stay alone with a psychiatric patient. Always have enough help to restrain a violent or potentially violent patient.
5. Do not confront any armed patient.
6. Look for medical reasons for the agitation and treat accordingly, i.e. head injury, hypoglycemia, drug overdose, intoxication, etc.
7. Protect yourself and others.

When to Use Restraint Procedures

The purpose of physical and chemical restraint is to prevent harm from occurring to the patient or others when all other reasonable methods have been exhausted. The use of physical restraints for patients who pose a threat to themselves or others is indicated as a last resort. Physical restraint should be preceded by an attempt at verbal control and only the least restrictive means of control necessary should be employed. Patient restraints should be utilized only when necessary and only in situations where the patient is exhibiting behavior that EMS personnel believe present a danger to patient or others. It is appropriate to use restraints when a patient is a danger to themselves or others as a result of a medical or psychiatric condition. If restraints are used, care must be taken to protect the patient from possible injury. When patient care and the provider's safety require the use of restraints, special precautions must be taken to reduce the risk of respiratory compromise.

Conditions that may result in a patient requiring physical restraint include, but are not limited to, substance abuse and psychiatric disorders. In addition, the combative behaviors requiring restraints may be associated with a syndrome of excited delirium posing an additional risk to the patient's health (Appendix C).

1. Use the minimum restraint necessary to accomplish patient care and ensure safe transportation.
2. Use restraints in a humane manner, affording the patient as much dignity as possible. Explain to the patient and family that you are restraining them so that they do not hurt themselves or someone else.

3. If law-enforcement or additional personnel are needed, call prior to attempting restraint. Physical *control and 'take-down'* of a combative individual should be the primary responsibility of police (unless waiting for their arrival would result in increased risk of injury to EMS personnel and safe retreat is not possible).

4. Restraint is not to be used on lucid, competent patients who are refusing treatment unless they are placed under a police hold. However, this procedure does apply to patients treated under implied consent.

5. A patient should only be physically restrained in a manner that is quickly reversible and allows for complete access to the patient.

6. Any patient placed under arrest should be transported with the arresting officer either in the transporting unit or following close behind for back up and/or support if needed.

Method of Restraint

1. All EMS personnel assisting in the restraint of a patient shall use personal protective equipment and universal precautions. Ensure sufficient personnel are present to control the patient while restraining him/her. USE POLICE ASSISTANCE WHENEVER AVAILABLE.

2. At no time should the actions of EMS personnel jeopardize the airway or respiratory effort of the patient, e.g. holding of the neck, chest restriction, or any other maneuver that would interfere with the life support needs of the patient.

3. Restraint equipment applied by EMS personnel must be either padded leather restraints or soft restraints (i.e. posey, Velcro, or seat belt type). All methods must allow for quick release.

4. The application of any of the following forms of restraint should not be used by EMS personnel:
   - Hard plastic ties or any restraint device requiring a key to remove.
   - 'Sandwiching' patients between backboards, scoop-stretchers or flat as a restraint.
   - Restraining a patience's hands and feet behind the patient (i.e. leg restraints)
   - Other methods or materials applied in a manner that could cause respiratory, vascular, or neurological compromise.

5. The patient must be positioned in a manner as to ensure adequate airway control and to allow for IV access.

6. Ideally, (if available), five persons should be involved in a coordinated take down of the violent patient each holding one extremity and/or the head.

7. As gently as possible, secure the patient to a backboard with secure restraints. (Be prepared to logroll immediately for vomiting.) (See illustrations in Appendix C)
   - Place patient face up on long backboard if at all possible.
   - Secure all extremities to backboard (4-point restraint.)
   - If necessary, utilize cervical-spine precautions (tape, foam blocks, or CID, etc.) to control violent head or body movements.
   - Place padding under patient's head and wherever else needed to prevent patient from further harm to self or restricting circulation.

- Secure backboard onto gurney for transport, using additional straps, if necessary, and be prepared at all times to logroll, suction, and maintain airway.

8. Consider whether placement of restraints will interfere with necessary patient-care activities or cause further harm. Therefore, avoid placing restraints in such a way as to preclude evaluation of the patient's medical status (airway, breathing, circulation). Monitor and chart the restrained patient's airway, circulatory and respiratory status constantly.

9. The patient must be checked and treated for any other medical or traumatic illness, i.e. hypoglycemia, OD, etc.

10. If providers are at risk of contamination by salivary and respiratory secretions from a combative patient, a protective device may be applied to the patient to help reduce the chance of disease transmission in this manner.

11. Document the patient's mental status, lack of response to verbal control, the need for restraint, the method of restraint used, the results, any injuries to patient or EMS personnel resulting from the restraint efforts, the need for continued restraint and methods of monitoring the restrained patient.

12. Restraint equipment applied by law enforcement (i.e. handcuffs, plastic ties, or leg restraints) must provide sufficient slack in the restraint device to allow the patient to straighten the abdomen and chest and to take full tidal volume breaths. Restraint devices applied by law enforcement require the officer's continued presence to ensure patient and scene safety. The officer should, if possible, accompany the patient in the ambulance. A method to alert the officer of any problems that may occur during transport should be discussed prior to leaving the scene. In situations where the patient is under arrest and handcuffs are applied by law-enforcement officers:
    - The EMS provider will monitor neurovascular status of hands.
    - Transporting patients with handcuffs behind the back is NOT an acceptable position of transport unless any other means of transport or restraint would put EMS personnel at risk of injury.
    - The patient should not be cuffed to the stretcher
    - A law-enforcement officer, with the handcuff key, shall accompany the patient in the ambulance if the handcuffs are to remain applied. If this is not possible, the officer shall follow by driving in tandem with the ambulance on a predetermined route.
    - A law-enforcement officer may elect to follow the ambulance in the patrol car if the patient has been restrained with restraints other than handcuffs

13. Restrained extremities should be evaluated for pulse quality, capillary refill, color, nerve, and motor function every 15 minutes. It is recognized that the evaluation of nerve and motor status requires patient cooperation, and thus may be difficult or impossible to monitor.

14. Document every 15 minutes or beginning and end if less than 15 minute transport. The medical incident report (MIR) shall document the following:
    a. The reason the restraints were needed
    b. The agency that applied the restraints
    c. The periodic extremity evaluation
    d. The periodic evaluation of the patient's respiratory status

15. ALTERNATE METHODS WITHOUT BACKBOARD.

    a.   Alternative methods such as stretchers and gurneys are only to be used when a backboard (which should be considered optimum) is not available.

    b.   (Monitor respiratory status very closely with these alternate methods.)

    c.   Each extremity is restrained to the stretcher. Cot straps must be in place.

    d.   Monitor and document reasons for applying restraints.

    e.   Monitor airway status, vital signs and neuro-circulatory status distal to restraints.

The Question of Prone or Hobble Restraint

Combative individuals in police custody will frequently be placed in a prone (on their stomach) or hobble position to ensure the safety of officers and others around them. As will be discussed in detail in Appendix B, there is no medical or research evidence that either of these positions compromises breathing or restricts the airways. However, they do make it more difficult to render appropriate medical care, so with the aid of police, EMS should transition the patient to positions best suited to accomplishing this goal: placed face-up, on a long backboard and secured with appropriate restraints, unless a medical condition requires another position (such as pregnancy which requires placement in the left lateral recumbent position to not compromise fetal circulation). <u>Patients should not be transported in the prone position unless necessary to provide emergency medical stabilization or required to assure officer and EMS safety.</u> EMS personnel must ensure that the patient position does not compromise the patient's respiratory/circulatory systems or does not preclude any necessary medical intervention to protect the patient's airway should vomiting occur. It is essential that police and fire/EMS cross-train to make the transition from police custody to medical restraints safe and efficient.

Chemical Restraint

Attempts to restrain the patient by conventional means will be attempted prior to considering chemical restraint (NOTE: As outlined in Appendix C, suspected Excited Delirium cases may require chemical restraint the moment the patient is physically immobilized). Because of the variety of chemical restraint protocols used by different agencies, we will not recommend any particular protocol here. Here are some essential principals:

1.   Do not administer a chemical restraint to a multi-system trauma patient.

2.   Watch and monitor for sudden respiratory collapse after physically and or chemically restraining an agitated subject.

3.   Monitor ECG and pulse oximetry, if at all possible.

4.   'Basic Life Support' (BLS) shall not transport chemically restrained patients.

5.   RSI and chemical paralysis should be used as a last resort to allow for patient/provider safety and emergency patient care based upon the severity of illness and/or injury.

APPENDIX B

The Question Of Positional And Compression Asphyxia
Gary M. Vilke, MD, FACEP, FAAEM

Background on Positional Asphyxia:

- The concept of "Positional Asphyxia" was originally based on research that had significant methodological flaws (Reay, et al 1988)
- The premise of positional asphyxia was that if you left a patient in a hobble restraint position, he would tire, go into ventilatory failure and then asphyxiate into cardiac arrest.
- The hobble position is defined as prone with hand cuffed behind the back and ankles restrained with a device that is then pulled up and tethered to the handcuffs leaving the knees bent.
- The original research and dozens of papers since have NEVER shown hypoxia (low oxygen levels in the blood) to develop in the hobble position.
- The original research and dozens of papers since have NEVER shown hypercarbia (elevated CO_2 levels in the blood) to develop in the hobble position.
- In fact, the only paper to report that the hobble position results in positional asphyxia, actually demonstrated that oxygen saturation levels IMPROVED in all subjects who were left in a hobble position.
- Subsequent studies evaluating obese subjects also have demonstrated that when left in a hobble position, they will not asphyxiate.(Sloane, et al 2014)
- All of these studies prove that people left on their stomachs in a hobble position will not die from asphyxiation, which includes both thin and obese individuals.

Best practices:

When encountered with a patient in a hobble restraint, certain assessments of a patient are critical and the documentation of the findings in the pre-hospital record is essential.

A. Assess the level of consciousness. Is the patient awake or not and is he verbal?

B. Assess perfusion. Is his skin color good and does he have a strong regular pulse?

C. Place on a monitor as soon as feasible and document first rhythm.

D. Place on pulse oximeter as soon as feasible and document O2 sat. If placing on a finger, make sure the hand is getting good perfusion through the handcuff if the O2 sat reading is low.

E. If the patient can be safely transferred to a supine position with approved 4-point restraints secured to the gurney – this is the optimal position as one has full access to the patient's airway and direct visualization of the face and access to the chest.

F. If the patient cannot be safely transferred out of the hobble position, attempt to transfer the patient in a lateral decubitus position on the gurney – preferably with the face and chest facing the EMS personnel to optimize monitoring.

G. Face down on the gurney in the hobble position is the least desirable position as the patient cannot be easily monitored or accessed if the physical status changes. If utilizing this position for transport, care must be taken to assure the airway is clear and not obstructed by sheets or the mattress.
   ***Despite all of the data supporting the safety of the hobble position, this is the position that will have the most scrutiny in a lawsuit if a patient deteriorates into cardiac arrest.

H. Ongoing monitoring and vigilance is important. The issue of medical concern is not the actual hobble position, as this is deemed physiologically neutral, but rather the concern is the underlying medical condition (drug induced or not) that required the patient to be hobbled in the first place.

I. These recommendations are meant to supplement, not replace, existing EMS protocols (blood glucose assessment, IV fluids, etc)

Background on Compression Asphyxia:

- The concept of "Compression Asphyxia" evolved after the theory of positional asphyxia was essentially debunked. (Chan, et al. 1997, Chan et al 1998)

- The premise of compression asphyxia was that a certain amount of weight is often placed on the back of an individual to get him into custody and handcuffed. Often this weight is multiple officers holding the person down with hands, forearms or knees. During this time period while the weight is being applied, the theory is that the subject would tire, not be able to breathe (ventilate), go into ventilatory failure and then asphyxiate into cardiac arrest.

- Research with up to 225 lbs of weight on the backs of healthy volunteers has not demonstrated physiological changes that would indicate that asphyxiation is likely with these weights. (Michalewicz, et al 2007)

- Studies with weights on the backs of normal subjects has also shown that cardiac output and blood pressure are not impacted.(Savaser, et al 2013)

- If an individual is alive, moving and breathing after the weight has been removed and then subsequently goes into cardiac arrest, the weight did not cause compressive asphyxia. *There is not a delayed asphyxiation*, it either happens while the weight is on or it does not occur.

- Even if the weight on an individual is so great as to restrict adequate ventilation, if the subject is breathing once the weight is removed, the person will breathe out the retained CO_2 and will recover. The effects of the weight are not lasting and a breathing individual will self-correct very quickly.

- It takes a great deal of weight, consistently placed over the ventilatory muscles of the back, for a significant length of time with essentially complete impedance of ventilation without breaks to breathe in order to theoretically cause a death due to compressive asphyxia.

- If a person is vigorously and repeatedly yelling or screaming, he is moving air in and out of his lungs and thus is not meeting the "complete impedance of ventilation" criteria and thus is not in a position at that time to cause asphyxiation.
   NOTE: That being said, other medical emergencies CAN present with the *sensation* that one cannot breathe, when in fact they are ventilating fine but are suffering from a myocardial infarction or ischemia, for instance. These patients should be carefully evaluated.

Best practices:

When EMS encounters a patient who had weight placed on him to get him into custody, certain assessments of a patient are critical and the documentation of the findings in the pre-hospital record is essential. Basically the patient will either be spontaneously breathing with a pulse, or not. If he is spontaneously breathing with a pulse, then he did not suffer from compression asphyxia and should be assessed and documentation should follow as per the "Best practices" for positional asphyxia (above).

If the patient is not breathing or does not have a pulse, treatment is basically standard advanced cardiac life support measures. Documentation optimally should reflect the events that led up to the cardiac arrest. Often EMS is present or staged within viewing distance of the event. If so, some of the following observations can be critically useful in evaluating the case for quality review or a subsequent legal action:

- How many officers where physically involved?
- Where were they located on the subject? (i.e. holding legs, holding head, knee on back, hands on shoulder, etc)
- How long was weight on the subject?
- Was the weight moving and shifting (did the subject arch up, roll over or was he just laying flat on his stomach)?
- At what point did the subject stop yelling in relation to the cardiac arrest?
- Was the change in status sudden or gradual over time?
- Was there weight on him at the time of the cardiac arrest and if so, how much?

Pearls:

Careful monitoring – you will likely be unable to prevent a patient who is suffering from Excited Delirium Syndrome from going into cardiac arrest. Additionally, rapid recognition and treatment is unlikely to change the ultimate outcome for the patient, but careful charting and documentation is extremely beneficial for subsequent legal actions that are likely to arise.

ETCO2 – If possible, document the earliest possible end tidal CO_2 level. Pre-intubation with bag-valve-mask is best if feasible, as this value if low or normal, will support that the individual did not asphyxiate, as CO_2 levels are high in patients who asphyxiated.

Careful accurate documentation with details as clear as possible. These cases in which there is a cardiac arrest often end up in litigation, so clear documentation of what was observed and reported with specific details is incredibly helpful in evaluating the case.

> **Appendix B: CAUTION**
>
> Medically evaluate the subject carefully, even if the person is vigorously and repeatedly yelling or screaming. It may be obvious that he is moving air in and out of his lungs and thus is not in a position at that time to cause asphyxiation – however other medical emergencies, like myocardial infarctions or ischemia can present with the sensation of difficulty breathing and should be considered during the assessment.

References:

Chan TC, Vilke GM, Neuman T, Clausen JL: Restraint position and positional asphyxia. Ann Emerg Med 1997;30(5):578-586.

Chan TC, Vilke GM, Neuman T: Reexamination of custody restraint position and positional asphyxia. Am J Forensic Med Pathol 1998;19(3):201-205.

Michalewicz BA, Chan TC, Vilke GM, Levy SS, Neuman TS, Kolkhorst FW. Ventilatory and metabolic demands during aggressive physical restraint in healthy adults. J Forensic Sci 2007;52(1):171-175.

Reay DT, Howard JD, Fligner CL, Ward RJ. Effects of positional restraint on oxygen saturation and heart rate following exercise. Am J Forensic Med Pathol. 1988 Mar;9(1):16-8.

Savaser DJ, Campbell C, Castillo EM, Vilke GM, Sloane C, Neuman T, Hansen AV, Shah S, Chan TC. The effect of the prone maximal restrained position with and without weight force on cardiac output and other hemodynamic measures. J Forens Leg Med. 2013 Nov;20(8):991-5. Epub 2013 Aug 30.

Sloane C, Chan TC, Kolkhorst F, Neuman T, Castillo EM, Vilke GM. Evaluation of the Ventilatory Effects of the Prone Maximum Restraint Position (PMR) on Obese Human Subjects. Forens Sci Int 2014;237:86-9. Epub 2014;46(6):865-72. Epub 2014 Feb 14.

APPENDIX C

A Multi-Disciplinary Response Protocol For Suspected
Excited Delirium Syndrome (ExDS) Incidents

By Lieutenant Michael Paulus (ret.)

Appendix C: Figure 1 – Excited delirium is a chaotic rage state

As discussed in detail in Chapter 49, Excited Delirium is a medical syndrome that is included within a general category: Chaotic Rage. It should not be incumbent upon either eyewitnesses or first responders to distinguish between excited delirium and other similar, equally dangerous forms of chaotic rage. The authors, therefore, recommend that protocols in your jurisdiction be coded for chaotic rage, with a clear understanding that this term encompasses excited delirium and other similar states, whatever the cause.

A Medical Emergency that Presents Itself as a Law Enforcement Problem

Deborah Mash, Ph.D., from the University of Miami Brain Endowment Bank, has called ExDS, "a medical emergency that presents itself as a law enforcement problem." It is clear from this statement that it takes a coordinated effort from various agencies to manage the challenges that present themselves when dealing with a patient in this chaotic rage state. When a plan is well set up, and inter-agency training frequent and effective, this integrated multi-disciplinary strategy fosters communication and respect amongst the various stakeholders and results in an effective team approach. This is in contrast to all-too-many instances where each of the responding parties acts independently, leaving some to pick up the pieces afterwards.

To effectively manage an individual in a suspected ExDS state depends on the cooperation of emergency dispatch, law enforcement, and Fire/EMS to get the right personnel on scene as quickly as possible. Fire/EMS personnel are the first who can actually help address the numerous medical issues that can lead to a sudden unexpected death of the ExDS patient. However, those in chaotic rage states also present the possibility of serious injury to first responders, particularly Fire/EMS personnel, who are not normally trained or equipped to protect themselves from violent assault. Law enforcement/corrections plays a supportive role to do three essential things: Capture, Control, and Restrain. Without this, FIRE/EMS will rarely get a chance to treat the medical emergency.

What follows is a highly effective protocol that has been used in Champaign County, Illinois since July 2008. Communities around the United States have adopted it in various forms. The primary focus is to get the patient to the emergency department as quickly as possible to give them the best chance for survival. The byproduct of this is a better working relationship between FIRE/EMS and law enforcement/corrections that translates into other areas in which they find themselves working together.

The Phenomenon of Excited Delirium: A Clinical Syndrome

In September 2009 the American College of Emergency Physicians put out the "White Paper on Excited Delirium Syndrome." The report stated, "Because of varied underlying medical conditions that may generate ExDS, there is also variation in the specific symptom cluster....The combination of delirium, psychomotor agitation and physiologic excitation differentiates ExDS from other processes that induce delirium only."[35]

A special report of ExDS was released in December, 2011 that was funded by the National Institute of Justice and conducted by the Weapons & Protective Systems Technologies Center at the Pennsylvania State University entitled, "Special Panel Review of Excited Delirium." The panel, made up of medical doctors, PhDs. and law enforcement personnel, looked at response protocols from around the country. The chair of Penn State's Department of Pharmacology, Dr. Kent Vrana stated, "I suspect there are going to be many pathways to [ExDS]. . . .There is not [necessarily] going to be 'a disease,' but it [(ExDS)] manifests itself as a syndrome,"[36] meaning that it will present itself as several clinically recognizable features, signs, and symptoms.

Based on my review of established research, as well as my own firsthand contact with several patients demonstrating the common behavioral signs and symptoms, ExDS can be viewed as "a metabolic freight train to death." All too often, the patient arrives at a point where their body has been compromised to such an extent that, even with expert medical treatment, they will not survive. Our primary focus, therefore, is to get the patient under physical control so that FIRE/EMS medical intervention can take place as soon as possible to avoid the "train pulling into the station."

The firefighter/EMS perspective, as is usual in medical crises, typically starts with an evaluation as to what is causing this behavior in order to determine how to treat it. Because of the extreme risk to self and others that these patients present, we must deal with the behaviors first, and *then* let the medical personnel figure out what might have caused them. In short, one must stop the behaviors and then control that metabolic freight train first. Otherwise, not only the patient, but first responders may be injured or killed.

From what is currently known, the most common precipitant of ExDS is stimulant drug abuse. Drugs like cocaine, methamphetamine, LSD, and PCP have been reported as the most common drugs ingested. Other substances, such as 'bath salts' (cathinones) and Spice (so-called 'synthetic THC') are increasingly figuring into such events.[37] Further down on the scale of frequency are mental health issues, predominantly schizophrenia and bipolar disorder. It is generally thought that patients who are non-compliant with their medication regimen are the ones most susceptible to ExDS. Dr. Gary Vilke, et al. wrote, "Less commonly, persons with new-onset psychiatric disorder, particularly those with manic or psychotic features, will present with ExDS."[38] Other precipitating factors include hyperthermia, meningitis, diabetes, alcohol-related delirium tremens, and head injuries, among many medical conditions. Even individuals on the autism spectrum in a 'meltdown' can manifest chaotic rage states, and appear to be acting like the ExDS patient who took stimulant drugs or has a mental illness.[39] Because it is impossible to diagnose such factors while under assault, or while the patient is in an extreme chaotic state, first-responders must address the behaviors first, the possible cause only ascertained later, once it is safe to do so.

The Role of the Telecommunicator

It is important to understand that the patient may be anywhere on the continuum of ExDS when first contacted—not everyone is necessarily "naked, sweating, and howling at the moon." They may be in the early stages of the process—confused, delirious and somewhat agitated. They could already be de-escalating on their own by the time first responders arrive (They can easily flare up again in an extremely agitated state, so first responders should do their best to initiate verbal control and de-escalation to assist the individual in restoring themselves to a calmer state).

It is essential that all telecommunicators be trained to identify the typical behavioral indicators present in a suspected ExDS incident. Gathering salient information from the caller, the telecommunicator can dispatch all of the needed resources to the scene early in the process. As telecommunicators are speaking with the reporting person or the law enforcement officer on scene, they should ask clarifying questions to be able to pass on to FIRE/EMS regarding the behavioral indicators of a suspected ExDS patient. For example, getting the estimated weight of the patient will assist FIRE/EMS, so they that can start to consider a possible dosage for sedation options available to them.[40]

Do Not Diagnose in the Street

It is unreasonable to require that either telecommunicators or law enforcement to be 'positive' that a person is in a state of ExDS. Emergency room physicians, who have been trained to look for the common presentation symptoms of ExDS, will definitely make a treatment plan based on their evaluation, but even this is uncertain. In fact, the only people that will know 'for sure' will be a medical examiner who understands the unique signs of an ExDS patient or Dr. Deborah Mash, Ph. D. and associates who, after testing of the patient's brain specimens, can possibly draw a clear determination. Both of the latter parties are involved after the patient has died. Therefore, law enforcement officers, telecommunicators, and even paramedics should not diagnose what is causing the behaviors that manifest as chaotic rage, but simply address them. The focus is to "err on the side of caution and cast a wide net" as Dr. Michael Curtis, M.D. from Wisconsin has said.[41] The goal is ensure that all ExDS patients receive treatment, understanding that you may respond to some who turn out to be other than true ExDS cases. However, in any such event, you will be dealing with an individual presenting in a chaotic rage state (Chapter X), so the behavioral indicators will be consistent, regardless of what the final diagnosis may be.

From First Contact to Aid Car—Getting the Patient Safety Under Control

Dispatch should send law enforcement along with FIRE/EMS at the same time to avoid the potentially fatal delay in getting the medical resources on scene. Furthermore, telecommunicators should send enough officers to make this possible, typically four to six officers for an effective capture with six an optimum number.[42] In situations where there are not that many officers on the scene, then competently trained FIRE/EMS can, and have, assisted in the capture of these patients. What is essential is that the law enforcement officers (and properly trained FIRE/EMS) have the restraints (handcuffs and hobbles), and are specifically trained on how to take control of a resistive patient. This topic will be discussed below when talking about "Multiple Officer Control Tactic" (MOCT).

If law enforcement arrives before FIRE/EMS, and the patient is not an immediate threat, it is suggested that they wait to make contact with the patient until FIRE/EMS arrives, something easier said than done. The crucial issue is that the more intense the patient's physical exertion, the more likely that they will pass the aforementioned tipping point into a complete metabolic crisis, and this very definitely includes struggling with first responders. This risk has to be balanced by the immediate threat to others, including the law enforcement officers, on whether or not to place hands-on the patient. It is strongly suggested that FIRE/EMS avoid making contact with the ExDS patient alone, but this, too, can be a challenge if the call was initially dispatched as a medical crisis, and they are the only ones on the scene before realizing the ExDS nature of the call.

Once Law Enforcement and FIRE/EMS are on scene, a quick plan of action should be developed so all of the first responders know what is going to happen. This can be as simple as the lead law enforcement officer or the team quarterback, designating who will capture the arms, who will take the legs, and what is available to them to take the patient down. (When it comes to takedown options, the conducted electrical weapon, CEW (Taser®), is one of the best options available). The law enforcement personnel will need to know if FIRE/EMS will sedate the patient as part of their ExDS sedation protocol. This all can be accomplished in less than a minute, and then law enforcement, with FIRE/EMS assistance if needed, can capture, control, and restrain, (followed by the latter sedating the patient if that is part of their protocol).

Some non-law enforcement personnel are understandably frightened of CEW devices, but this is not warranted, when the devices are used properly. It is important to understand that unless FIRE/EMS gets between the wires, the risk of getting shocked is minimal. Even if there is a shock, it is not nearly what the patient is experiencing either. A concept that is taught to law enforcement is to 'cuff under power.' This means that while the patient is experiencing neuromuscular incapacitation (NMI) and has limited abilities to resist, law enforcement should move in, put hands on and start the capture process.[43] Once the initial charge is delivered, the officers should be in a position to better control the patient. FIRE/EMS should be behind or off to the side of the law enforcement officers when the CEW is deployed so as to avoid exposure to the device. Additionally, if a CEW is used, FIRE/EMS will potentially need to address any collateral injuries from the patient falling.

Once the patient is on the ground, face down, law enforcement will move to control the patient's arms and legs. FIRE/EMS must understand the law enforcement will need to put the patient in a prone position for a short time in order to get control of the patient for this process. The patient, once restrained, will be placed in a supine position for FIRE/EMS to treat the patient.

The best and safest tactic to physically control a combative patient is one of skeletal isolation, that I call the "Multiple Officer Control Tactic" (MOCT). The main concept behind the MOCT is to keep the patient under control, even though they may be manifesting a superhuman level of strength and lack of response to pain. This is done not by putting weight on their back, but by limiting their ability to use their limbs to resist. The arms are secured by keeping them above the shoulder line by the use of abduction, and using the knee of one of your legs to support your wrist while pinning the shoulder of the patient to the ground. This also limits the patient's ability to bite the law enforcement or FIRE/EMT controlling the arms. The legs must also be secured, or the patient can keep moving him/herself and the officers around. Not only might they escape, but it also makes it less secure for FIRE/EMS to attempt sedation. Preferably two law enforcement officers or FIRE/EMS personnel move the patient's legs apart, so they are less able to brace against the ground and use strength. Weight is placed down by the ankles by lying on the legs. This limits the strength of the patient's legs. This also presents FIRE/EMS with options for intramuscular injection options in the buttocks or upper thigh.

To better control the patient prior to any sedation by FIRE/EMS, law enforcement/corrections secure each of the patient's wrists with a chain-link handcuff. Holding onto the handcuff is more secure than holding onto a sweating or possibly bleeding wrist while ensuring that body substance isolation (BSI) precautions are taken against pathogen-infected body fluids. Once a handcuff is on each wrist, the person in charge of the capture and control process will advise FIRE/EMS that they can now administer the approved sedation option (it should not be attempted until the patient is secure in this manner). Communication between law enforcement and FIRE/EMS not only makes it safer for those involved, but also helps achieve the capture, control, sedation, and restraint in the shortest time. This is not only beneficial for the patient, but also for the first responders who are working to get the patient into the ambulance and on the way to the Emergency Room.

The decision to sedate the patient is ENTIRELY that of the paramedic, based on their training and direction from the EMS Medical Director—law enforcement officers have absolutely no say in this matter. If FIRE/EMS determine that the patient is not appropriate for chemical restraint, they must communicate that to the law enforcement personnel as early as possible, so that they can move right from controlling the patient to restraining them in multiple sets of handcuffs.

After the sedation (or if there was no sedation given), the patient should be restrained by law enforcement with handcuffs and a hobble restraint. I recommend a minimum of three sets of handcuffs be placed on the patient, depending on their size, in a so-called 'daisy chain.' More than three sets may be required to be able to turn the patient to the supine position for transport. The patient should have their hands down by their sides to make it easier for the FIRE/EMS to get an IV started or other medical procedures initiated. The patient's legs are secured by a hobble restraint to keep the patient from kicking law enforcement, FIRE/EMS, and Emergency Room personnel. IMPORTANT: The patient should not be hog-tied as that would make it difficult for FIRE/EMS to actually treat them. The hobble is tied to the end of the backboard the patient is placed on before the restraints used by FIRE/EMS (spider straps or other restraining straps) to secure the patient to the backboard are applied. Once the medical restraining straps are applied, law enforcement will assist in getting the patient onto the gurney and then into the ambulance for transport. Law enforcement should NOT remove their cuffs and hobble until arrival at the ER where the hospital's leather restraints can be provided (if the patient is not sedated). Even when the patient is sedated, the number of cuffs used through this daisy-chain method will give FIRE/EMS room to work.

Appendix C: Figure 2

The focus must remain that this is a medical emergency—that takes precedence over any criminal issue. The criminal charges can wait, the medical emergency will not!

A law enforcement officer should ride in the back of the ambulance with FIRE/EMS to assist as needed. The adage "handcuffs on, cop rides along", is very appropriate for these situations. Law enforcement can also communicate any pertinent information about the patient to FIRE/EMS that will help with treatment options. Were FIRE/EMS need to have the handcuffs removed for treatment purposes during transport, the law enforcement officer will have a handcuff key. The way to restrain the patient would be to secure the cuffs to the gurney: one hand above their head and the other hand down below their waist to prevent them from sitting up. This prevents the patient from being able to sit up and possibly head-butt someone in the ambulance.

Law enforcement is also there to observe the actions of FIRE/EMS with the patient while en route to the hospital. Law enforcement can then also advise Emergency Room personnel of any relevant facts about the situation and the patient they may need for treatment purposes.

The Question of Field Sedation

On the question of sedation options for possible ExDS patients, EMS Medical Directors get comfortable with certain medications based on their track record and clinical efficacy. Some of the common drugs used for field sedation include midazolam (Versed®), lorazepam (Ativan®), ziprasidone (Geodon®), and haloperidol (Haldol®). There have been successes and failures using each of these drugs when attempting to control the chaotic rage of an ExDS patient. The decision to sedate the patient must be is founded on a well-structured evidence-based protocol. The Fire/EMS personnel must have options to handle the complexity the ExDS patient presents.

There have been several field studies showing the benefits of the use of the dissociative anesthetic, ketamine (Ketalar®) as a potential sedation option. Ketamine is considered by a growing number of EMS Medical Directors as the best available drug for this situation as it has a rapid onset of action, it is highly effective in a single dose, it preserves airway protective reflexes, it is IM injectable, it is reliable in its effects, it supports heart rate and blood pressure, and it has a very good safety margin.[44], [45], [46] Ketamine has been used in the Champaign County Sedation protocol with excellent results. (NOTE: Ketamine is brought up here as a consideration by the EMS Medical Directors as an alternative and does not mean that a protocol cannot be created that does not use ketamine).

At the Emergency Room

Once the ambulance arrives at the hospital, it is imperative that a core body temperature is obtained as soon as possible. One of the most common physical presentations of ExDS is hyperthermia. Unfortunately, if the patient has not been sedated and is still highly agitated—which causes the body temperature to continue to rise and the effects to exponentially grow as well—the core temperature may not be checked in favor of dealing with the other issues. If the patient dies at a later time and no temperature was obtained, it is evidence that is lost forever.

Dr. William Weir, MD of Carle Foundation Hospital in Urbana, Illinois, an Emergency Room Physician and the EMS Medical Director for Arrow Ambulance, has proposed a series of tests that should be considered by ER physicians when an ExDS patient has been brought into their facility. Dr. Weir suggests the following tests for addressing the many medical issues an ExDS patient presents:

- Initial vital signs including rectal temperature
- 12-lead EKG
- Venous blood gas
- Serum lactate
- CBC and CMP
- Serum Ethanol
- CK (creatinine kinase)
- 10 drug urine, urine HCG (if applicable)
- Chest x-ray, head CT without contrast
- Continuous pulse oximetry
- Continuous heart monitoring

The point of these tests is to address the multitude of problems that the ExDS patient can present. The ER physician will need as much information from the FIRE/EMS and law enforcement on what they had to deal with on scene in order to get a full clinical picture. This includes any medications and dosages that were administered: both on scene and on the way to the ER.

These tests also become evidence in the case that this vulnerable patient dies, an ever-present possibility in these cases. Unfortunately, the autopsies in ExDS incidents often do not reveal a clear anatomic reason for the death. It is then left to others to make their case as to what led to the person's death without much medical or scientific evidence, leading, all too often, to baseless accusations against law enforcement or others.

It is important for the Medical Director of each ambulance company to be brought into the protocol development process as early as possible. The Medical Director is the one who will make the final decisions on what the protocol will look like—they must understand what the paramedics are facing in the street or in the correctional center with ExDS patients. The Medical Director should understand the restraint procedures used by law enforcement, what options there are for field sedation of the suspected ExDS patient, and what types of testing should be done on these patients should they arrive in the Emergency Room alive.

FIRE/EMS should prepare early with a good well-structured evidence based protocol as well as an online protocol involving medical control through radio communications with an Emergency Department physician for further orders or repeat dosages.

In any process that addresses the multitude of problems that FIRE/EMS faces in an ExDS incident, there must be a quality control process to review these incidents to gauge their effectiveness. There may be unexpected things that occur in the field, and a simple review process can address these situations to avoid future problems. Drug effectiveness is also one that most Medical Directors will want to know about in case a change in dosage or medication is warranted. Remember the adage: "Don't train to get it right, but train so you can't get it wrong." This can only happen when the protocol has been well thought out and trained with all of those that will be involved in the process. Mutual aid training has benefits that cannot be measured when it comes to these 'low frequency/high liability' incidents.

ExDS in Correctional Facilities

ExDS incidents that occur in a jail or correctional center present particular challenges, even though the general protocol is the same.[47] The first issue FIRE/EMS will face in jail situations is the ability to get into the facility and safely to the patient, something that can be dependent on communication between FIRE/EMS and the facility as well as the staffing available to assist.

One advantage in such situations is that correctional staff may have a more detailed medical history of the patient, possibly including a mental health history, as well as any recent drug use that they are aware of when the patient was brought into their facility. The telecommunicator, who will be dispatching the FIRE/EMS units to the scene, should be included in such communication. It is imperative that they receive accurate information on who the patient is, where in the facility the incident is taking place, where FIRE/EMS will gain entry, and who will get them to the actual scene.

Some smaller correctional facilities are not necessarily staffed at sufficient levels to fully handle the capture, control, and restraint of the patient/inmate. This may necessitate other resources—deputies or other law enforcement personnel—who are called upon to assist the correctional staff. The capture tools available to the correctional staff are generally similar to what law enforcement personnel use. Many correctional facilities have trained personnel that are used for cell extractions or takedowns. These personnel may use CEWs or other tools to gain rapid control of the patient. It is suggested that FIRE/EMS (and law enforcement, if they will be part of the protocol for a specific institution) train with Correctional staff, just as with law enforcement, so everyone is competent with the capture and control process. Correctional staff may decide to keep the patient locked in their cell or other area that can be secured until FIRE/EMS arrives, similar to a situation in the community where law enforcement officers contain as best they can until FIRE/EMS arrives. This is again based on the understanding that struggling against the force of restraint might increase the metabolic demand on the body. If correctional staff leaves the patient in a secured area until FIRE/EMS arrives, this can potentially lessen the physiologic stress on the patient. Of course, this is contingent upon the situation. If the patient presents an active threat to other inmates or other staff, it is a better and safer option to get control of the ExDS patient/inmate as quickly as possible rather than waiting for FIRE/EMS.

Even with sufficient staff to assist in the capture, control and restraint of the patient/inmate, there may be other obstacles to care in a correctional environment: for example, the actual location of the incident. Is it in a cell? This might present issues with space for the correctional staff along with FIRE/EMS to be able to get to the patient/inmate, and still have enough space to work. The area involved may have items that could become weapons should the ExDS patient get them. The point is that even though this is a 'secure' facility, the environment itself could be a very 'insecure' one in which to deal with an ExDS patient. This underscores the necessity of clear communication and cross-training amongst the correctional staff and FIRE/EMS to prepare for confronting an ExDS patient in a correctional setting.

Summary

ExDS is a medical emergency that has presented itself as a law enforcement/corrections problem, one that, on the medical side, law enforcement/corrections are not trained or equipped to handle alone. FIRE/EMS are the first resource that can start to deal with the multitude of medical issues that are driving this "metabolic freight train to death."

Stimulant drug abuse is the most frequent cause for these behaviors, but it is important to understand that it is not ALWAYS a drug abuse cause. Mental illness, delirium tremens, hyperthermia, meningitis, autism, and other pathological issues can also be the cause for these behaviors. It is not necessary that FIRE/EMS personnel diagnose the cause, but rather deal with the immediate behaviors to stabilize the patient and get them to the emergency department as quickly and safely as possible.

Communication amongst all of the stakeholders is critical in getting the resources to the scene as quickly as possible. This should be followed by clear communication amongst the first responders to safely and effectively capture, control, and restrain the patient.

FIRE/EMS must have the necessary medical options to treat the ExDS patient, and best practice, therefore, includes sedation options. These will be based on a well thought out, evidence-based protocol. This protocol must be trained often enough so that it "can't be done wrong." ExDS are generally low frequency, but high liability occurrences, so the FIRE/EMS personnel must train often enough to be aware of how this is handled when it does occur.

Law enforcement/corrections need to 'stay in their lane,' fulfilling their responsibility to get the patient under control as quickly as possible. This will most likely necessitate putting the patient into a prone position long enough to get control. Once this is accomplished, the patient MUST BE placed into a supine position, with enough restraints applied, so that FIRE/EMS can begin the appropriate treatment. Once the patient arrives at the Emergency Room, the Emergency Department staff must know what types of medical testing are suggested to treat the complex issues facing these patients. This can not only help the patient survive, but it also may be vital evidence of the dire physical condition the patient presented to the first responders.

The collateral benefits of law enforcement/corrections training and working with FIRE/EMS in these incidents can have a huge benefit in other areas. The communication and respect for each resource's expertise pays off when they are involved in other situations involving mutual aid.

This "template" can be modified to fit the resources available to your area. Remember: the medical emergency takes precedence over any criminal issues or even a diagnosis.

If you would like to contact Michael to discuss this information, he can be contacted at Michael@michaelpaulustraining.com.

Lt. Paulus would like to acknowledge the assistance and input of Dr. William ("Brad") Weir, MD and Mr. Chuck Gipson in the development of this material.

Dr. Weir, MD, FAAEM, FACEP is a board certified Emergency Physician at Carle Foundation Hospital in Urbana, IL, and EMS Medical Director for Carle Regional EMS in east central Illinois. He is a former Paramedic, EMS Instructor, Flight Physician, and a veteran of the US Army National Guard and Air National Guard. His work email is william.weir@carle.com

Mr. Chuck Gipson, BA, NREMT-P, CCP, has been a Paramedic for 20 years, he is the Quality/ Education Manager for MEDIC EMS in Davenport, IA. He is the Co-Chair Medical Committee and Board of Directors for the John Deere Classic, and System Evaluation Quality Improvement Sub-Committee Co-Chair Iowa Department of Public Health. His work email is gipson@medicems.com

Multiple Officer Control Tactic (MOCT) – An Illustrated Guide

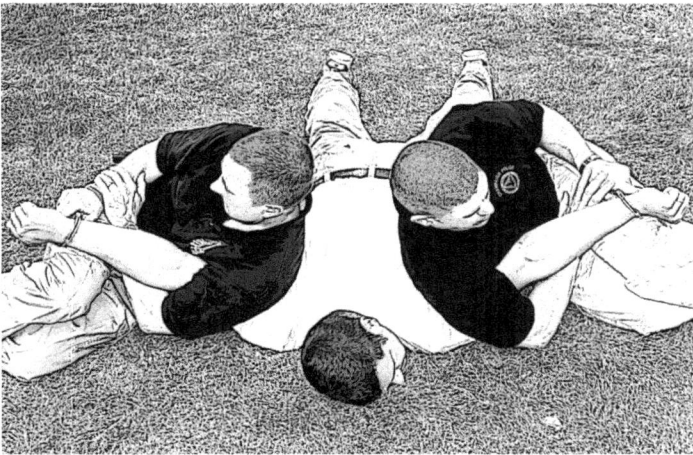

Figure#1- (Pin#1) Patient's arms are above the shoulder line with the officer's armpit on top of the shoulder. Patient's arms are controlled by officers by use of "figure four" along with a chain-link handcuff. Patient's arms are raised by using the officer's outside leg. Weight is kept off the patient's back to isolate the patient's shoulder.

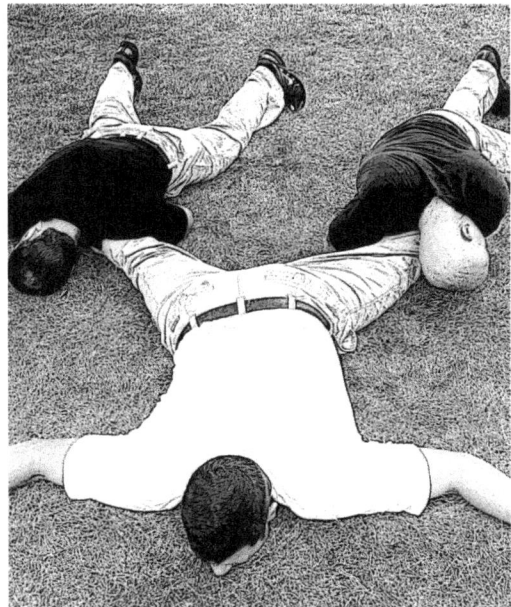

Figure#2- (Pin#2) Patient's legs are moved out from the centerline of the body to limit their power. Officers wrap the patient's leg with their arms and tuck the heel under the armpit on the outside of their body. Weight is kept low towards the patient's ankles.

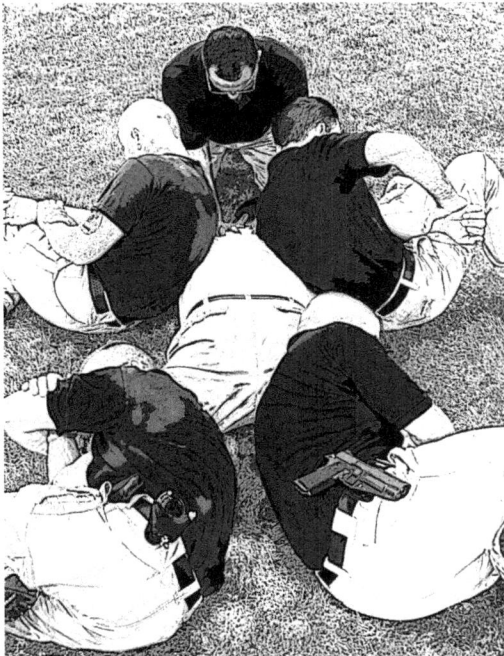

Figure#3- (Pin#3) Skeletal isolation is maintained by having two officers on the arms, two officers on the legs and then one officer at the patient's head. The officer at the patient's head is pushing down on the patient's trapezius muscles and monitoring the patient's status. This can be achieved by as few as three officers.

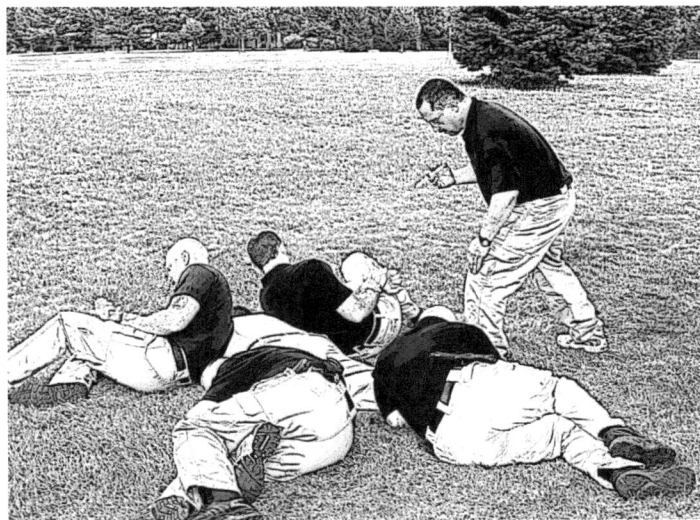

Figure#4- (Sedation#1) - EMS IM injection is achieved after the "quarterback" has confirmed that the arms and legs are controlled enough to allow EMS to approach the patient. EMS will move in from the sides which allow better access to buttocks or upper thigh of the patient.

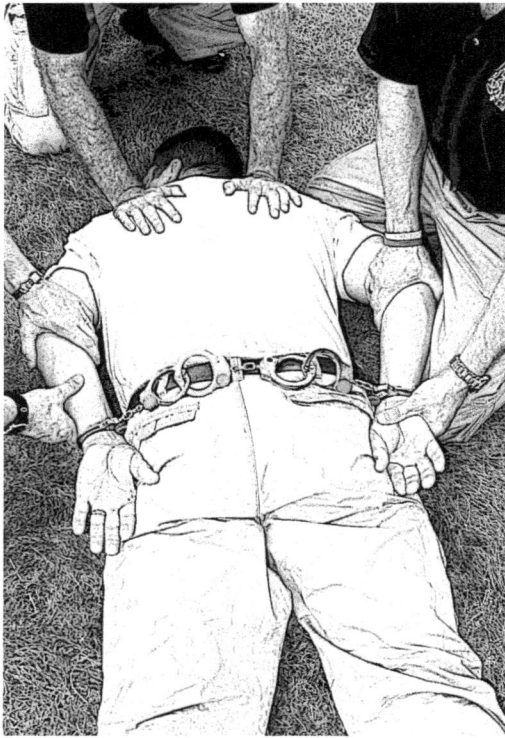

Figure#5- (Cuffing#1) - Once sedation has been given, officers will bring one arm behind the back at a time and apply at least three sets of handcuffs in a daisy chain configuration to allow the patient to be turned to a supine position. This will allow EMS to access the arm to establish an IV if warranted.

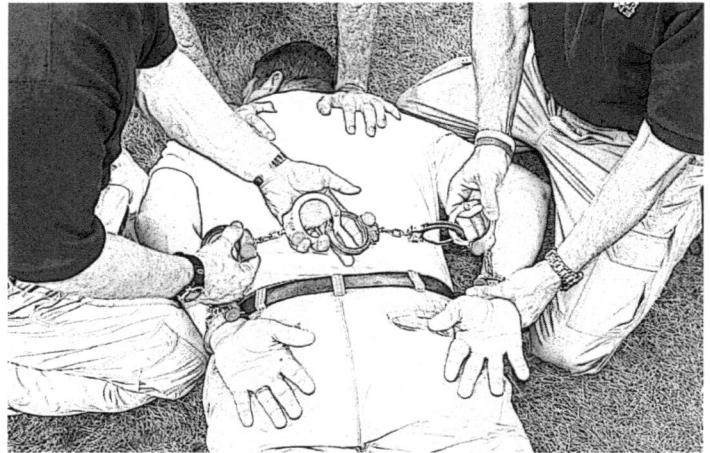

Figure#6- (Cuffing#2) - If the subject is larger, then four or more sets of handcuffs should be applied so that the patient can be placed in the supine position.

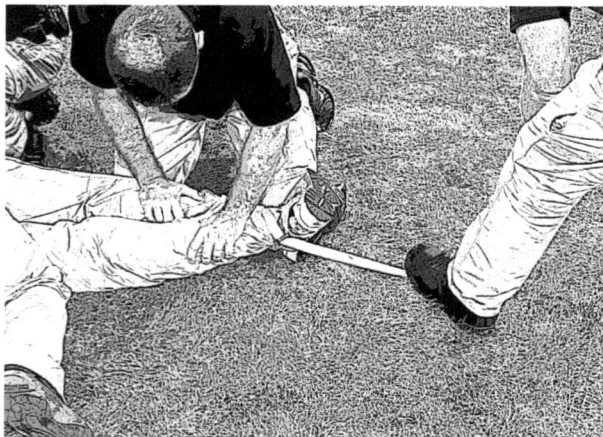

Figure#7- (Cuffing#3) - The patient's legs are brought together, ankles crossed if possible, then the nylon hobble is applied and pulled away from the patient. The other officer holds the patient's legs to keep them secured.

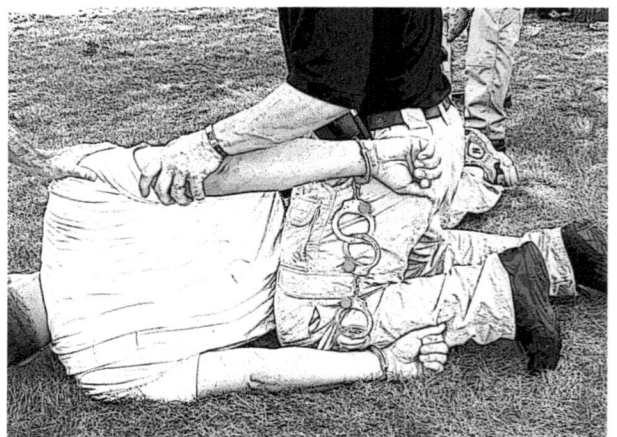

Figure#8- (Recovery#1) - If EMS is not on scene when the patient is captured, the officers are advised to place the patient in the left recovery position until EMS arrives on scene. Sedation can still be administered in this position.

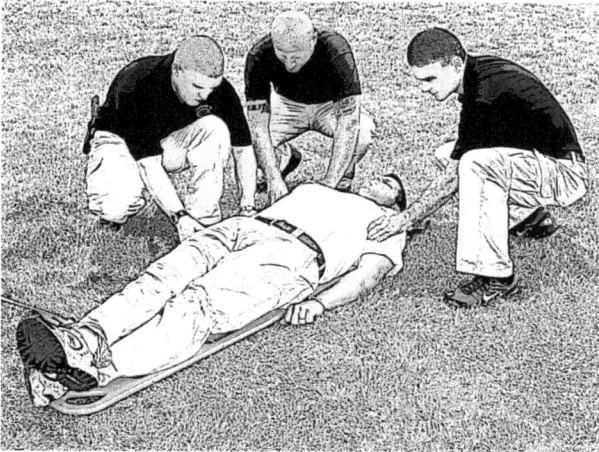

Figure#9- (Backboard#1) - The patient is placed on top of the backboard with the series of handcuffs under their back. This starts to limit the patient's ability to resist.

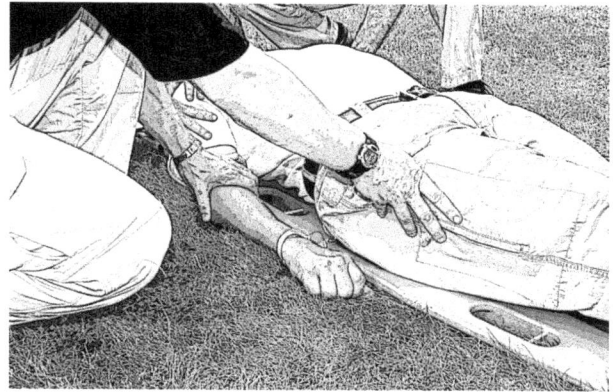

Figure#10- (Backboard#2) - Close-up showing patient on top of handcuffs while on top of the backboard.

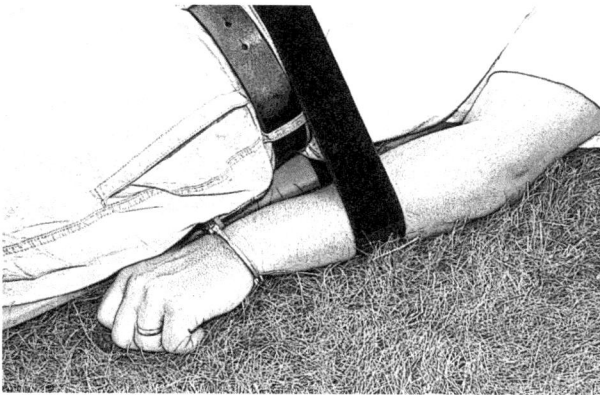

Figure#11- (Backboard#3) - Close-up of patient's arms while handcuffs are under the body and spider straps are applied. Notice that an IV could be started while in this position.

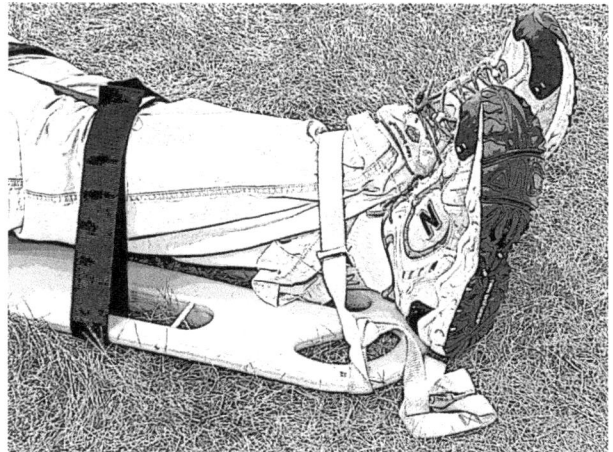

Figure#12- (Backboard#4) - Close-up of patient's legs secured to the backboard using the spider straps and the nylon hobble tied to the end of the backboard.

Endnotes

[1] This is the authors' best estimate derived from a number of articles in trade journals on this subject.

[2] United States Department of Transportation National Highway Traffic Safety Administration *EMT-Basic: National Standard Curriculum*

[3] HIPAA Privacy Rule and Sharing Information Related to Mental Health. http://www.hhs.gov/ocr/privacy/hipaa/understanding/special/mhguidance.html Unnecessary sharing of information between non-essential providers may lead to a violation of HIPAA and other patient privacy issues.

[4] Some dispatch centers purge their records of contacts after a certain period of time. This is a serious mistake—an incident of violence that occurred several years previously is still relevant to the safety of first responders at a later time. One of the authors is aware of a case of this nature where the lack of records was a contributing factor in an individual's death in a subsequent encounter with law enforcement. They had no idea of his past history of serious aggression because the call center kept records only for six months.

[5] DeBecker, Gavin, *The Gift of Fear*, Dell Books. (1999).

[6] Amdur, *EVERYTHING ON THE LINE:* Calming and De-escalation of Aggressive and Mentally Ill Individuals on the Phone *A Comprehensive Guidebook for Emergency Dispatch (9-1-1) Centers*, Edgework Books. (2011) www.edgework.info

[7] Amdur, Ellis, *SAFE HAVEN:* Skills to Calm and De-escalate Aggressive and Mentally Ill Individuals: 2nd Edition *A Comprehensive Guidebook for Personnel Working in Hospital and Residential Settings*, Edgework Books. (2011) www.edgework.info

[8] Amdur, Ellis & Cooper, William, *GUARDING THE GATES:* Calming, Control and De-escalation of Mentally Ill, Emotionally Disturbed and Aggressive Individuals *A Comprehensive Guidebook for Security Guards*, Edgework Books. (2011) www.edgework.info

[9] Amdur, *Safe Haven*, Ibid.

[10] First responders experience trauma somewhat differently from victims of violence. Unlike the latter, they have voluntarily walking into a dangerous situation. They accept this possibility as a liability of their job. The trauma may involve having to witness what others have done, engendering a feeling of helplessness. Other traumatic experiences involve feelings of guilt, either justified or not, in not helping or saving someone. For these reasons, an effective therapist must grasp that a first responder's trauma is associated with a particular kind of helplessness—that of someone who expects, and almost always is able to help and make things better. "I didn't save a life" is a very different trauma from "I thought I was going to lose my life." The effective therapist must understand both.

[11] Ekman, Paul. *Emotions Revealed*. New York: Times Books, Henry Holt and Company. (2003).

[12] You will sometimes see the same thing with people for whom English isn't a first language.

[13] Arieti, Silvano. *Interpretation Of Schizophrenia. 2nd ed.* New York: Basic Books. (1974).

[14] Delusional stalkers, the subject of this section, are quite rare. The majority of stalkers are not suffering from a major mental illness. Other major categories of stalkers are:

   a. Relational stalkers. This is often an extension of a controlling or violent relationship. The stalker either keeps tabs on his or her partner, or pursues them once they have left.

   b. Obsessive stalkers. The obsessive exhibits a hyper-focus on the victim, not necessarily to kill or even harm, but always to control. This stalker can be well-aware that the victim does not desire contact, and may be afraid of or hate him. But just as the germ-obsessed obsessive MUST wash his hands 50 times, despite *knowing* that they are clean, the obsessive stalker has to have the attention of his victim.

   c. Terroristic stalker such a patient may certainly have been in a relationship or be obsessed with his victim. There is also considerable 'ego' involved; this stalker's psychological energy focuses on himself rather than the victim. A true predator, he is doing something he enjoys. Why? Because he can: either for amusement, or because the victim, in some way, offended him (revenge).

[15] Our thanks to Aaron Fields of the Seattle Fire Department for another version of this intervention.

16 An actual incident—the engineer was killed trying to jump clear when the manic person wrecked the train.

17 Researchers note that a mixture of alcohol and cocaine is particularly dangerous, as the body synthesizes them together into a new substance, cocaethylene. See: http://jpet.aspetjournals .org /content/274/1/215.abstract

18 Allen, B., & Bosta, D. *Games Criminals Play: How You Can Profit by Knowing Them*. Berkeley, CA: Rae John. (1981-2002).

19 Hare, Robert. *Without Conscience: The Disturbing World of the Psychopaths Among Us*. New York: Guilford, (1999)

20 According to New Jersey Lawman website (http://www.njlawman.com/2002_line_of_duty_deaths.htm), there were 120 line-of-duty deaths in 2009. This included homicide, vehicle accidents, line-of-duty illness, and accidental weapons discharge. According to a police suicide prevention website (http://www.policesuicideprevention.com/), there were 143 police officer suicides in 2009. Our thanks to Dr. Sherwin Cotler for drawing our attention to these statistics.

21 http://www.cdc.gov/ViolencePrevention/pdf/Suicide_DataSheet-a.pdf

22 In this last case, the perpetrator was a former surgical nurse. Her cuts were perfect—doctors stated that they could see her internal organs beneath the sheath of fascia. Once in the hospital, she had to have her arms restrained, because she would rip out the stitches, reopening the wound.

23 One of the writers does recall a para-suicidal individual who cut her wrists on repeated occasions. One sheriff deputy, after a background check, informed her that he was aware that she was a doctor and knew exactly how deep and where to cut. He promised to arrest her if there was another such incident. She moved to another state.

24 Please note that this type of plan for 'frequent fliers' is individualized. You cannot impose this plan on a similar person in your area, but you can use it to develop your own, one suitable to the person about whom you are concerned, and congruent with the resources (and laws) in your community. That's why you need to get together with all the 'players' involved both in the 'frequently-in-crisis person's' treatment and in the emergency response system that is now part of their life, and figure out the best, tactically and humanly sound plan for that person.

25 After that twelve-year period, she again cut herself after some kind of emotional stressor. By chance, my co-developer of this plan was in the ER on another case. She sat down with her, kindly (but 'distantly') pointed out that this type of behavior had never helped her, and she didn't need to do it anyway. People wanted to talk with her when she was having trouble, not attend to her wounds. She then praised the woman for being so 'good' about this over the last twelve years and said, "I know you can do it again." She's not been seen by emergency personnel since.

26 Levinas, E. *Ethics and infinity: Conversations with Philip Nemo*. translated by Richard Cohen, Pgh, PA: Duquesne University Press. (1985).

27 De Becker. G. (1999). Ibid.

28 You may have a different 'count' for your inhale/pause/exhale. Find the ideal pattern that allows you to breathe smoothly, without strain.

29 See the work of Dr. John Gottman of the University of Washington for a detailed discussion of contemptuous silence and stonewalling. Gottman's books mostly concern couples, but the principles he describes can be applied to any interpersonal relationship.

30 The authors owe a debt for some of the basic information in this section to a form of training called Professional Assault Response Training (PART), thanks to a workshop one of us attended approximately 25 years ago. We have made major changes in their basic 4-part schema, as well as adding a significant amount of new data. Therefore, our approach is quite different, and it shouldn't be confused with PART's procedures.

31 Dr. Sherwin Cotler, Ph.D. Written communication

32 Salter, Anna, author of *Predators: Pedophiles, Rapists and Other Sex Offenders: Who They Are, How They Operate and How We Can Protect Ourselves and Our Children*. New York: Basic Books. (2004)

33 Edited to cite the Washington Law for the reader – Murphy, J. K. 2014

34 The information in this section is derived from information from Clark County, Washington; Walla Walla County, Washington; Snohomish County Fire District; Spokane County, Washington EMS;

35 American College of Emergency Room Physicians (ACEP), "White Paper Report on Excited Delirium Syndrome: ACEP Excited Delirium Taskforce," (2009), p. 10

36 Hughes, Lt. Colonel Edward L. (ed.), "Special Panel Review of Excited Delirium," pub., Weapons and Protective Systems Technologies Center, Pennsylvania State University, (2011), pp 14-15

37 Murray BL et al. , "Death Following Recreational Use of Designer Drug 'Bath Salts' Containing 3,4,-Methylenedioxypyrovalerone (MDPV)," *Journal of Medical Toxicology*, (2012)

38 Gary M. Vilke, et. al., "Excited Delirium Syndrome (EXDS): Defining Based on A Review of the Literature," *The Journal of Emergency Medicine* (2011), p. 5

[39] Ho, Jeffrey D. MD, Paul C. Nystrom, MD, Darryl V. Calvo, MD, Marc S. Berris, JD, Jeffrey F. Norlin, AS, Joseph E. Clinton, MD, "Prehospital Chemical Restraint Of A Noncommunicative Autistic Minor By Law Enforcement," *Prehospital Emergency Care* (2012), Early Online: 1–5

[40] Amdur, *EVERYTHING ON THE LINE, Ibid.* [Appendix, Suggested Response Protocol for 9-1-1 Concerning Suspected Excited Delirium Incidents — by Michael Paulus] pp. 207-214

[41] Dr. Michael Curtis, M.D., personal communication

[42] DeMaio, Theresa and Vincent, *Excited Delirium Syndrome: Cause of Death and Prevention,* CRC Press, (2005), p. 34 - "The recommended minimum number of medical personnel to physically restrain an individual in excited delirium is six."

[43] Individuals in ExDS states will not respond to CEW as an aversive stimulus as ordinary combative individuals will, and instead of giving up, will reinitiate combat as soon as NMI ceases. 'Cuffing under power' enables officers to subdue and restrain the patient when they are physically incapable of resisting.

[44] Ho, Jeffrey D. MD, Stephen W. Smith, MD, Paul C. Nystrom, MD, Donald M. Dawes, MD, Benjamin S. Orozco, MD, Jon B. Cole, MD, William G. Heegaard, MD, MPH, "Successful Management Of Excited Delirium Syndrome With Prehospital Ketamine: Two Case Examples," *Prehospital Emergency Care* (2013), Early Online:1–6

[45] Burnett, Aaron M. MD, Joshua G. Salzman, MA, EMT-B, Kent R. Griffith, RN, EMT-P, Brian Kroeger, PhD, Ralph J. Frascone, MD, "The Emergency Department Experience With Prehospital Ketamine: A Case Series Of 13 Patients," *Prehospital Emergency Care* 2012;16:1–7

[46] Scheppke, Kenneth A. MD* Joao Braghiroli, MD† Mostafa Shalaby, MD‡ Robert Chait, MD§ "Prehospital Use of IM Ketamine for Sedation of Violent and Agitated Patients," Retrieved From http://escholarship.org/uc/uciem_westjem

[47] Amdur, Ellis, Michael Blake and Chris DeVillenueve, *SAFE BEHIND BARS: Communication, Control, and De-escalation of Mentally Ill and Aggressive Inmates.* Edgework Books, (2013), www.edgework.info

ABOUT THE AUTHORS

Ellis Amdur

Edgework founder Ellis Amdur received his B.A. in psychology from Yale University in 1974 and his M.A. in psychology from Seattle University in 1990. He is both a National Certified Counselor and a State Certified Child Mental Health Specialist.

Amdur has trained in various martial arts systems since the late 1960's, spending thirteen of these years studying in Japan. He is a recognized expert in classical and modern Japanese martial traditions and has authored three iconoclastic books on the subject, as well as one instructional DVD.

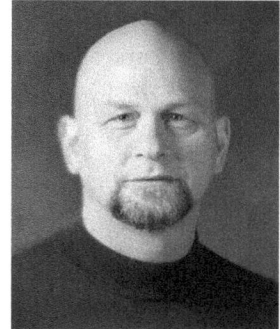

Since his return to America in 1988, Ellis Amdur has worked in the field of crisis intervention. He has developed a range of training and consultation services, as well as a unique style of assessment and psychotherapy. All are based on a combination of phenomenological psychology and the underlying philosophical premises of classical Japanese martial traditions. Amdur's professional philosophy can best be summed up in this idea: the development of a patient's integrity and dignity is the paramount virtue. This can only occur when people live courageously, regardless of the circumstances, and take responsibility for their roles in making the changes they desire. He has authored and co-authored a number of books on the de-escalation of aggression, like this one, specific to those in various professions. Please refer to Amdur's website (www.edgework.info) for a complete list of his books.

Ellis Amdur is a dynamic public speaker and trainer who presents his work throughout the United States and internationally. He is noted for his sometimes outrageous humor as well as his profound breadth of knowledge. His vivid descriptions of aggressive and mentally ill people and his true-to-life role-playing of the behaviors in question give participants an almost first-hand experience of facing the real patients in question. For further information please see Amdur's website: www.edgework.info

John K. Murphy

JOHN K. MURPHY, JD, PA-C, MS, EFO, retired as a deputy fire chief after 32 years of career fire department service, managing all areas of fire department operations and management positions. His past fire and emergency medical experience has been as a paramedic/firefighter for more than 20 years; paramedic program director, chief fire officer, chief of training, emergency operations chief and health and safety officer. Mr. Murphy lectures and writes on issues related to fire law and management. Mr. Murphy was a US Navy Corpsman serving with the US Marines.

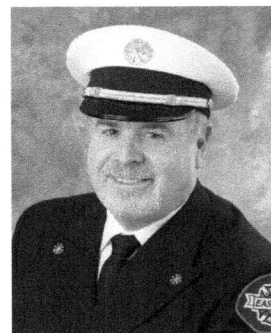

Mr. Murphy is an attorney with the Murphy Law Group, focusing on employment practices liability, training safety, employment policy and practices, forensic evaluation on fire and EMS operations, internal investigations, and as a subject matter expert in pre-hospital EMS and fire operations, consulting on risk management for private and public entities. He also has experience in family law, contracts, non-profit incorporations, mediation and internal investigations.

He is the Vice President of M2 Resource Group, Inc., a consulting company specializing in Fire and EMS legal and operational issues and a Physician's Assistant with a focus in urgent, emergency, occupational and pre-hospital medicine medical care. Mr. Murphy is the author of Legal, Political & Regulatory Environment in EMS, a Prentice Hall educational publication.

Mr. Murphy has a Juris Doctor (JD) from Seattle University School of Law; Masters of Science (MS) degree in education and Bachelors of Science (BS) in Paramedicine from Central Washington University and graduated from the University of Utah School Of Medicine, Physicians Assistant Program (MEDEX) and is an Executive Fire Officer Graduate. He is a licensed attorney in Washington and New York, a member of the bar associations in Washington, King County and New York. He is a member of the Association of Fire Service Attorneys; National Society of Executive Fire Officers; International Association of Fire Chief's; U.S. District Court Western District of Washington and legal counsel for the International Society of Fire Service Instructors (ISFSI), and an adjunct instructor for the University of Florida Fire and Emergency Services program.